D0938744

Ruth Rakoff

When My World
Was Very Small

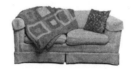

A Memoir of

FAMILY,

FOOD,

CANCER

AND MY COUCH

Random House Canada

COPYRIGHT © 2010 RUTH RAKOFF

All rights reserved under International and Pan-American Copyright
Conventions. No part of this book may be reproduced in any form or by
any electronic or mechanical means, including information storage and
retrieval systems, without permission in writing from the publisher, except
by a reviewer, who may quote brief passages in a review. Published in 2010
by Random House Canada, a division of Random House of Canada Limited,
Toronto. Distributed in Canada by Random House of Canada Limited.

www.randomhouse.ca

Random House Canada and colophon are registered trademarks.

Library and Archives Canada Cataloguing in Publication

Rakoff, Ruth
When my world was very small : a memoir of family, food, cancer and my
couch / Ruth Rakoff.

Issued also in electronic format.

ISBN 978-0-307-35817-2

1. Rakoff, Ruth. 2. Breast—Cancer—Patients—Biography.
3. Breast—Cancer—Patients—Family relationships. 4. Breast—Cancer—
Treatment. I. Title.

RC280.B8R35 2010   362.196'994490092   C2010-901395-6

Design by CS Richardson

Printed in the United States of America

2 4 6 8 9 7 5 3 1

For Tommy, Micah, Amit and Safi
My world big and small

—

And for Scott Sellers
My champion

KING SOLOMON FELT that his most trusted minister, Benaiah, was becoming too full of himself and needed to be humbled. Knowing that Benaiah could not possibly succeed, Solomon challenged him to find a magical ring that had the power to make a sad person happy and a happy person sad. Benaiah set about searching far and wide for this magical ring to no avail. Just before he was about to admit defeat and return to his king empty handed Benaiah came upon an old jeweler and asked the question he had asked so many times before. "Have you by any chance heard of a magic ring that can make a happy person sad and a sad person happy?" The old man reached in his bag and handed Benaiah a plain gold ring with an inscription. Delighted, he returned at long last to King Solomon and with great pride presented him with the ring. The king took the ring and reading the inscription realized that Benaiah had succeeded. On the ring was written "This Too Shall Pass."

Jewish Folk Tale

1

Where's Roof?

I T IS SPRING. The sun shines in the window and on good days bathes me in optimism. I sit lengthwise on my couch, my back propped against the armrest by an array of multicolored throw cushions, my legs extended and swaddled in the red, orange, purple, green, yellow quilt that begged me to take it with me when I passed it in the department store. *I belong with you*, it screamed, and I had to agree that it could not possibly find such kinship in another home. *Color. Color will help me find my way. My own red, orange, purple, green, yellow road back.* Its sequins glint at me as I sit with my notebook on my lap, pen in hand, spilling myself onto the lined pages, hour upon hour, day after day, searching for fragments of myself beyond grief, fear, worry. *I used to belong to the world I see beyond my couch. There must be a void of specific size, exact Ruth volume, a void that, if only I can find it, I will be able to reoccupy. My rightful place.*

These past seven months I have traveled to dark dark places. My journey in breast cancer has taken me beyond any borders I had previously known and deposited me here, here on the threadbare velvet, faded mustard yellow couch in the south-facing front window of my house. I am unrecognizable both to myself and to others. I have lost so much of myself along the way that when my young friend Rebecca comes to visit and I answer the door, she asks, "Where's Roof?" I'm working on the answer.

Growing up in the age of macramé, batik, tie-dye and other hippie crafts, I remember making multicolored candles. We would cut off the top of a cardboard milk carton, fill it with ice cubes and pour in paraffin that we'd melted in one of my mother's hijacked cooking pots. The hot wax would melt the ice cubes, leaving holes to be filled with another color of wax once the first color hardened. *I am full of icy holes. I must make something hot to fill the holes. I don't expect to be able to recreate the old me—I only hope to recover some of my previous solidity.*

The postal carrier delivers the mail. I wonder what he thinks of the woman in the hat, sitting on her couch day after day. Sometimes I want to bang on the window and explain that I've been sick. I am not lazy. I have in the past contributed to society. I used to leave my couch, and I even had a job. I want him to understand that I am in recovery and that is the reason I sit on my couch all the time. Why do I care what the mailman thinks about me? I'm so caught up in myself that it doesn't occur to me that he probably has no thoughts about me at all or what I'm doing on the couch.

I find the scratching of my fancy fountain pen on the paper of my dollar-store notebooks both soothing and amusing. The irony of how life catches up with one—every experience, every seemingly meaningless choice—is not lost on me. My pen, a special edition Montblanc, given to me by my father because I do not lose things, because I can be trusted to take care of such a ridiculously expensive object, glides along my pages with ease. And yet, while I still have this pen I was given many, many years ago, I have lost myself.

I write longhand because I cannot type. As a know-it-all teenager in need of a makeup credit, I registered for a night-school typing class. I justified my absence from all but the first and final classes by convincing myself that if I never learned to type, I would never have to suffer the presumed boredom of being a secretary. (Although, ironically I turned out to be such a fabulous waitress that employers were always reluctant to promote me for fear of losing my incomparable skills as a food schlepper.) Since a passing grade in typing did not require any degree of actual proficiency, I smugly believed that I had played the system to my advantage and dodged the secretarial bullet. I didn't give much thought to the fact that, much like driving a car or doing the laundry, typing is a life skill. One I still don't really have. Now, when I have to communicate using a keyboard, as in e-mail, I muddle through, but I'm certain that my hunt-and-peck two-finger dance on the keys significantly lowers my IQ. I am less stupid and faster with a pen and paper, so I sit and spend my time filling notebooks.

It feels as though I'm weaving an intricate tapestry with my ink, picking up loose threads and attaching new ones. I am trying desperately to make my recent journey fit; to draw upon the sum of my parts to recreate my whole. I am not looking for meaning or understanding necessarily, but for integration of the new me with the one that came before. I drive my couch slowly, carefully steering my pen through uncharted territory. It is not a strictly linear journey.

At night, after my children are asleep, I climb the stairs to my bedroom and settle myself under the covers next to my husband of more than twenty years. I do not want to be touched. I have not yet found peace in my body, which has betrayed me and been violated and brutalized by knives and needles and toxins. I cannot give away what I do not possess. Instead, I clutch my notebooks and read to Tommy, who patiently sits next to me in bed with his laptop and types my stories. Through my words, the words with which I am finding my way back to myself, I let him in. It is an act of the utmost intimacy.

As I read, I listen for the voice I once heard as mine. I work to steer clear of the overly sentimental, maudlin voice that I'm feeling and yet believe to be the epitome of weakness, sucky-ness, vulnerability. *Be funny*, I think, as I read aloud to the clickety-clack of the keyboard—but I do not feel funny. *Be bold. Be confident.* But I am not. Sometimes, my memories emerge as though they belong to someone else; as though the stories are not mine to tell. Has my vision been altered permanently by recent events? Have I lost accurate hindsight, precise history? *Could that be me free-floating in the middle of the South Pacific Ocean without fear or a sense of mortality? I recognize Tommy in my memory, long and lean and young and beautiful, a mane of hair snaking loose around his head as he floats belly-up to the sun. But the image beside him is blurred, unrecognizable. I cannot seem to conjure up the me that could act with sufficient abandon and confidence to trust that the water, and the world, would keep me safe.*

I test out different voices hoping that they might remind me of what my own voice sounded like before it was dislodged. Like a drowning person, I search in vain for air with which to fill my lungs. I gasp and begin again in a different voice—perhaps this one my own.

As a gift for my father's fiftieth birthday, my mother hired Mr. Ogaki the gardener to plant fifty rosebushes at the front of our house. Dad's rose garden. Much was made of this as the gift for "the man who had everything." And to be sure, he did have a great deal: a successful career in psychiatry, a beautiful home, three children of whom he could intermittently be proud, and a wife who was not only a respected family physician but also an outstanding homemaker and hostess.

Everything? I thought. *Really? Everything?*

A birch tree with boughs that wept and vivid green seed pods that littered the flagstone walkway every July. A carefully thought-out Japanese garden of low-lying shrubs, glinting rocks and pebbles, and a sand pit that no one ever played in. And above it all, a vast, aging maple canopy with its floating helicopter pilots that drifted down to land in the crevices between the white quartz stones at its imposing base. White cylindrical pillars flanking the subdued yellow front door. To the far right, beyond the garden, the asphalt driveway, matte against the glossy black of the garage doors . . .

Hardly everything, I thought. *Nice, but not everything.*

Later, when I was older and less sheltered, I understood how not to be so literal. For most of the world there was no Mr. Ogaki, no gardens, no frivolity. Dirt was for growing food. My father had his own path leading up to his own door. Not one, but two trees. Stones and wood and asphalt, and sand to ignore in summer and snow to shovel in winter. A garage door that opened and closed with the press of a button. And a wife who might not have promised but indeed delivered a rose garden. Everything!

Tommy and I also have everything. We have grown up together. We met when he was fourteen and I was sixteen at socialist Zionist summer camp. We didn't become a couple until some years later, but even that was more than two decades ago. We have history. I sometimes worry that according to some grand, cosmic plan we have exceeded our allotted time together in this life, having met so young. Perhaps there is only so much good life to go around and we have used up our quota, overdrawn on our happiness account, so to speak. Maybe that's why I got sick. Maybe it is somebody else's turn to have it easy, normal, uncomplicated.

But that is my cancer voice talking. It speaks from fear and apprehension, from sadness and grief. It is my fragile voice, not my resilient voice. I know I still have that one too. We all do. It's what makes life possible. When things become difficult, abnormal, complicated, we must declare, proclaim, announce. Don't whimper. Don't whine. Don't crumble.

In many ways, one would be hard-pressed to find a more conventional couple than the two of us. Both church and state—our church being a rabbi—legally married us. We have a house with a nice big mortgage, a car with a lot of years and mileage, three kids. But those are just the right-angles of the box that is our life together. To the outside eye we look settled in our average, "normal" world. We seem lucky. And in fact we *do* have everything.

Including cancer.

Arrgh! There it is—that voice I'm trying to suppress. It pops up unexpectedly. Must I accept it as part of me, or can I reach down my own throat, pull it out and quash it?

It has been an evolution rather than a metamorphosis, this ordinary life we lead. As youngsters we were social-ists, feminists, adventurers, risk takers. We would be different than our parents. We had no interest in average or normal or status quo. Armed with my degree in litera-ture—a fierce weapon to be sure—and with Tommy schooled as a jazz musician, we moved across the world. After almost four years of living and working in Tel Aviv we traveled in the Far East for seven months before returning to Canada. We ventured off the beaten track with courage and abandon. Our thoughts were not of creature comforts, nor cushy beds, nor soft toilet paper, nor uncontaminated food or water. We were invincible, immortal. I want to find my immortality, but I fear that is lost forever.

While we were living abroad, my mother sent me a cartoon she had clipped from the newspaper. It was a drawing of a woman whispering into a telephone, and in the background, sitting on a couch in the next room, were a young woman and a long-haired, grubby looking young man. The caption read: "Help, Police! My daughter wants to marry a musician!" It was funny in part because my parents loved Tommy the musician from the get-go. He was talented, smart, kind and handsome, and posed a distinct possibility of introducing height into our vertically challenged gene pool. Nonetheless, they worried about us. They worried about us being so far away. They worried that we'd never earn a decent living. They worried about us because we are their children.

At the same time that Tommy and I moved to Israel, my younger brother David decided to put his college education in Japanese studies to the test and departed for a stint in Tokyo. My parents worried about him also. They worried for the same reasons. They worried for different reasons. They worried about him being far away. They worried about him being alone. They worried about him because he is their child. When after only three months he returned to Canada with Hodgkin's lymphoma, I don't know if they worried more or less about Tommy and me in Israel. And, despite David's subsequent complete recovery, I believe they have never stopped worrying about him in a different way than they worried about us—until now.

Cancer is not normal. Is worrying about cancer normal? I worry a lot these days. I hate the me who worries about cancer and dying. I hate the me who gets anxious about getting enough sleep so I don't feel sick, so I don't worry that maybe the cancer is back. I want to find the me who can tell the difference between tired and sick. Where's Roof?

Our decision to leave Israel was not an easy one. I remember speaking with my father on the phone across the miles and lamenting the predictability and stability of Canada in comparison to the vitality, the excitement, the precariousness of Israel. "Perhaps one day you will be happy for stability, for normal," he said.

After our return to Canada I changed careers like some people change hairstyles, never really finding anything I was passionate about. (*I must remember not to look for myself in my résumé. I am unlikely to be there.*) Tommy went back to university to study computer science while playing in a rock band and waiting to be discovered. Then our first son, Micah, was born and just when it looked like we were finally settling down, off we went to California so Tommy could work for a dot-com think-tank. Then, back to Toronto, two more boys, Amit then Safi—and here we are at run-of-the-mill family of five.

My boys need me back. I used to be a real mother. I used to be the one who tucked them in at night and folded their socks and shouted at them to tidy their rooms and do their homework. I haven't shouted at my children in such a long time. I don't have the energy. I wonder if they remember what I sound like when I shout. Note to self: Shout at children more often.

Despite our days in the socialist youth movement, the hours spent debating equality and feminism and my relentless efforts to prove that I was physically up to any job a man could do, I have become a "domestic diva." Though we sometimes took a round-about route to get here, "conventional" is more or less what we've become. We have adopted what can be called "traditional" roles in our relationship. Tommy helps, but I have always been responsible for home and family. Compared to most men of my father's generation, Tommy is like a male Martha Stewart. He does dishes, makes beds, changed diapers, takes out the garbage and more. My favorite saying is "Tommy can do anything I set my mind to." He is willing and able, as long as I am there to give instructions. "Can you make me a list of the things I need to do," he says. And armed with said list he is unstoppable.

Since we met so young and I am two years his senior, I have often teased that I found Tommy when he was just tiny and grew him and grew him. Along the way, though, I forgot to teach him how to cook. This is funny because Tommy is six foot five. It's *not* funny because he really never learned to cook. He would no doubt take great offense at this claim and argue that it is not entirely true, but for the purposes of storytelling, it is essentially true. Who plans the meals, does the grocery shopping, and virtually all of the cooking? Me. And our traditional roles don't stop there. Who makes social arrangements, doctors' appointments and plans extracurricular activities? Who makes sure all family members have clean clothes that more or less fit and don't have too many holes? Who makes sure our various schedules are coordinated with regard to arrivals, departures and mealtimes? Me, me, me.

Not wonderful me. Not powerful me. Just me, because over time it has become my job to run our family. Tommy's contributions to our family are no less important, they are just different.

But I have not done any of these things for a long time now. Not since my journey in cancer began. I have not planned meals or grocery shopped or cooked. I have absolutely no idea what is in my fridge. I do not drop off children or pick them up and I have only a vague idea where they are supposed to be at any given time. These

WHEN MY WORLD WAS VERY SMALL

days I only go to my own doctors' appointments. And I'm pretty sure all the boys are sharing socks and underwear, because the laundry hasn't been properly sorted in months.

I grew up in a neck-up household. Cerebral pursuit, not physical, was the modus operandi of our family. For the most part, I was alone in my interest in athletics and outdoor activities and was practically accused of family treason for corporeal involvements. As Rakoffs, we sparred with our tongues, engaged in conversation, banter, repartee, not ball games or races. Our bodies were appendages, more apt to cause harm or accidents, at least in my father's nervous perception. Whenever my brothers and I would get physical, as even Rakoff children were inclined to do on occasion—a game of tag or hide-and-seek considered the height of athleticism—my father's refrain was, "That's a recipe for disaster!" It was as though this brilliant man had absolutely no comprehension of running or jumping or moving swiftly. Ordinary childhood activity that didn't involve books or art supplies frightened him. The notion of "a recipe for disaster" both intrigued and bewildered me. After all, a recipe was something one used to get things "just right." Was there a way to get a disaster "just right"? Why would you bother with a recipe for something you didn't even want? Okay, so maybe I wasn't the sharpest Rakoff in the drawer.

But when faced with the prospect that my illness and treatment would put me out of commission for an extended period of time and Tommy would have to assume responsibility for all my usual territory, I had a rare jolt of insight. What we needed was a crisis plan, a management strategy—a *recipe for disaster*. We needed to call upon all our collective resources, our friends, our families, our community, our past and our present to help us through.

And now, all these months later, having made it over the pinnacle of the crisis with the help of so, so many, I need to concoct a different kind of recipe. A recipe to grow myself and expand my world beyond this faded mustard yellow couch in my sunny window.

2

Tumbling Turtles

I T WAS A BEAUTIFUL, SUNNY DAY at the end of August with a faint whiff of autumn in the air. My boys and I were all on our bikes as we wound our way through the neighborhood and I delivered each child to a different friend's house.

"Where you off to?" my neighbor Barb shouts from across the street.

"Mammogram," I shout back.

"Oooh, the squish."

I give her a ring of my bike bell and a wave and head off for my annual squishing. Still an ordinary day.

———

Before cancer entered my personal space, I was Yertle the Turtle at the very top of that big pile of turtles—I was queen of all that I surveyed. Well, perhaps not queen, so much as maid, secretary, personal assistant, tutor and overseer of all other administrative aspects of my life and the lives of my husband and children. I was involved with committees. I had meetings to attend. I knew who had homework, music classes, swimming lessons, and how everybody would get there and back. I was in tune with what was going on in my friends' lives, their children's lives, and in my community. I knew what was in my fridge and what was on my grocery list and what to do about all of it. I ran businesses, taught classes, managed staff, advised families, even took responsibility for other people's children.

With cancer, my world shrank. My turtle tower came tumbling down, and suddenly control of all things, from the organization of my pantry and linen closet to the choice of how much of my breast would be amputated, was gone. In fact, the only choice remaining was, Do I say yes or no to potentially life-saving treatment? And they were blunt, the medical professionals. It suited me fine in some ways. I was by no means stoical. I cried through most of my doctors' appointments, but no one lied to me or candy-coated the reality. And, although the truth was harsh, I needed to know it.

There were niceties and attempts to create the illusion of choice regarding my treatment, but none of them fooled me, at least not for long. Cancer does not invite you to attend. It doesn't even tell you when the party is. It just shows up and, if you're lucky, after subjecting yourself to hellish treatments, it goes away. But, you never know. It could come back. You don't get to choose or control that either.

"Would you like to come back in? We need to get some more pictures," the radiology technician says after seeing something suspicious on my mammogram.

Sure, I'd love to come back in. I figure I'm already dressed for the occasion in my thin cotton hospital gown which, whether done up in front or in back, does not allow one to maintain even a modicum of dignity. Of course, I can't think of anything better than coming back in and for the second time today having you sandwich my breast between two cold sheets of Plexiglas and squeezing it till my flesh is spread as thin and wide as pancake batter on a well-oiled griddle.

Or maybe, no thank you, I'd really like to put my clothes back on and get out of here like last year and the year before. And thank you very much for providing me with this routine medical check that I am so grateful to submit to once a year in order to be reassured that all is well.

Oh, you weren't really asking.

"That's great! Now, if you'd like to step into this room over here, we'd like to get an ultrasound as well."

Really? An ultrasound? You make me feel so special. I've never gotten this kind of attention at my mammogram before, but again I'd rather be going now. I'm finding it a bit chilly in this thin little gown, and while I don't want to sound rude or ungrateful, your attitude is beginning to elevate my angst beyond my comfort zone.

Again, not really a question, I suppose.

"We'd like to get a biopsy of this thing. What's your schedule like in the next week?"

As though my schedule has any bearing on anything.

Now I'm starting to clue in. Maybe it's my tears that have cleared the view. I no longer determine what my schedule is. I fit in. I don't choose. I say "yes" and "okay." I get it.

Yes please, the sooner the better.

Leaving the hospital that day, I still believe that I have some control. Before I have even unlocked my bike I phone my GP on my cell.

"Hi, it's Ruth Rakoff calling. I just wanted to let you know that something showed up on my mammogram," I say with a matter-of-factness I don't feel. "They'll be faxing you a report and a request for you to book a biopsy. I thought I should give you a heads-up so you can do that ASAP." Just taking care of business.

I dial Tommy.

"Hi. Ya, I'm just leaving the hospital. So, uh, something unusual showed up on my mammogram and we're going to do a core biopsy and investigate further," I say, trying to make it sound like it was my idea. "We'll just have to wait and see what happens."

I say goodbye, unlock my bike and ride off to pick up my kids, still choosing which route I take, still controlling how fast I pedal, still setting the pace, the tone, the outcome of the instant.

3

Sedatives and Sandwiches

A FRIEND ONCE TOLD me how her very proper
Protestant grandmother avoided conflict. Any-
time something verging on unpleasant, disturbing or off-color came up in conversation, Grammy would
offer up sandwiches. The list of verboten subjects was
long, befitting a woman of her upbringing and generation. Everything from the disturbing news that a lady
had ventured out without panty hose, to the eventual
decay of the world as she knew it could be skirted skillfully with a tight smile and an offer of sandwiches. The
decline of civilization and propriety, to the point that
one's daughter could speak about matters of a personal

nature, like sex, or money or divorce, kept Grammy very busy in the kitchen.

"Who wants sandwiches? I have tuna, cheese, egg salad . . . ?"

As someone who more often than not is inclined to tell it like it is, face the uncomfortable head-on and point out the emperor's lack of clothes, I found tales of Grammy side-splittingly hilarious. My amusement made light of an old lady's worries—I didn't understand that she was building herself a fortress cemented with butter and Miracle Whip. Grammy was arming herself with tuna, cheese and egg salad. As long as there was Wonder Bread and spreadable filling, Grammy could pretend that all was right in the world.

Over time, "who wants sandwiches, I have egg salad . . ." became, in our household lexicon, code for *I am about to talk about something difficult that could cause tension, or other discomfort.* It was kind of like those jokes that begin "I have good news and bad news."

"Who wants sandwiches? I have tuna, egg and I got fired."

"Who wants sandwiches? Tuna, egg, the toilet overflowed."

When I called Tommy after the suspicious discovery on my mammogram, I did not offer him sandwiches. There was nothing about tuna, cheese or egg salad funny enough to deal with this situation. And no one offered sandwiches to me.

What I was offered were drugs. Until then, I had no idea who was stashing what, but suddenly it seemed as though everybody had access to something or other, and they were all willing to share. My family doctor was first in line.

On the morning after my mammogram she called. "I've requisitioned a biopsy," she said. "Until then there is nothing to do but wait. I can write you a scrip for sleeping pills if you want."

"No thanks. I think I'll manage," I said. I wasn't ready to give in to potential negative outcomes just yet. I have always suffered from sleep problems, and at that point I believed that I could cope with more of the same, at least until I had real cause for alarm.

One week later, running on adrenaline, almost no sleep or food and with Tommy's hand held firmly in my viselike grip, I faced my core biopsy. It is a procedure in which, guided by an ultrasound image, the physician uses a tool that looks and sounds like a gun with a long, hollow needle attached, to harvest a cylinder of flesh from the suspicious region of one's body. The procedure is done under local anesthetic—an offering I didn't refuse—and while it is by no means pleasant, it doesn't hurt.

I wept through the whole thing. Full-blown heaving and sobbing bringing me close to hyperventilation. I am not that person. At least I had never before been that person. This was the new me. I was so overwhelmed and agitated that I managed to make myself dizzy lying on the table.

"I think I'm going to pass out," I said.

"That's not possible while you're lying down. Just try and calm down, dear," the nurse suggested a little patronizingly. "Try to slow down your breathing. Deep breath in—two, three, four—now let it out slowly—two, three, four."

But I could tell she thought I was being hysterical. Even *I* thought my behavior was melodramatic, but it was beyond my control.

"Your doctor will call you with the results in a week to ten days," she informed us as she ushered us toward the door. "Don't worry."

But, truth be told, I was desperately worried. I had been feeling unwell for about six months: first it was just a cold that I couldn't seem to get rid of, followed by a bad case of bronchitis from which I emerged even weaker. I had gone to my doctor and told her that I knew it was just a cold, just bronchitis, but I was feeling worse. So, we had embarked upon a slew of medical investigations, but thus far had turned up nothing substantial. Nevertheless, I was sure there was something sinister lurking within me. When we got home from the biopsy, a procedure that took all of an hour, I experienced an exhaustion befitting serious physical exertion, and passed out on the couch.

When I woke up, Tommy had made me an egg salad sandwich.

Within a few days, my physician parents were next to offer me sedatives. Though they were not in the habit of prescribing for family members they felt some exceptions applied. Tommy must have told them about my Oscar-worthy performance through the first of what would turn out to be many procedures. Finding ourselves alone for a moment, my father approached me in his well-worn therapist's mantle.

"You are understandably distressed," he said, taking my fingers in his warm, dry hands. "You needn't suffer, you know. I can give you a few Ativan and write you a prescription for some more." His tone of understanding and sympathy was the kind for which mental health professionals are mercilessly satirized.

Desperately holding back tears, my lifelong Pavlovian response to my father's offers of support, I said, "I'll let you know."

"I understand your concern, but it isn't helpful to be so overwhelmed," my mother said in what anyone who didn't know her might interpret as a critical tone. "Take a couple of Ativan for tonight and you can get a prescription filled in the morning."

I knew it was her way of coping, not the direct order it sounded like.

"That's okay," I replied.

Having no real news yet, either good or bad, I still felt confident that I could go it alone.

That weekend, Tommy, the boys and I met my brother David in Buffalo. We had originally asked him to join us for our annual get-together with our friends Jordanna and Rob and their boys, believing there might be fodder for David's journalist-at-large essay writing in Rob's army surplus business. As it turned out, the timing of the trip was perfect. Though David has lived in Manhattan since he was about seventeen years old and is loath to leave for any reason not work related, family crisis draws him like a magnet. A pre-arranged convergence in Buffalo under the guise of "research" prevented David from having to make a last-minute trip to Toronto in the heat of the moment of possible crisis. Nothing like a solid *maybe* to get everybody worked up into an impotent frenzy.

David, who has worked hard to perfect his neurotic New Yorker persona, is never without his security Xanax. I don't believe he uses it very often, but just knowing that it is close at hand, should the need arise, seems to limit the circumstances where the need arises. He carries it around like a good luck charm, in a pocket-sized tin of after-coffee mints.

"I have Xanax. You should take it," David offered barely on the heels of "hello." "I don't know how long I've been carrying this one around, but it couldn't hurt."

"Thanks, but no thanks," I said.

"You're an idiot. Just take it," he said, combining the roles of concerned brother and pusher.

"I'm trying not to worry until I have something concrete to worry about," I said with false bravado.

"Fair enough," he said, backing down.

"I wish I had something stronger than booze to offer you," Jordanna, our hostess for the weekend in Buffalo, lamented. "But I don't, so what would you like to drink?"

I am not a drinker. Though I like an occasional beer, overindulging gives me a headache. But suddenly, getting a headache was a risk I was willing to take.

"Anything in copious quantity," I replied.

Over the next few weeks, I would take to drink like a fish to water—or at least, like someone with something significant to worry about. With drink somehow I could pretend that it was all about the party. Pills, I feared, would strip me of my comfortable cocoon of delusion.

A week after my biopsy, the abstract possibility of cancer became a fact. My family doctor called me on

Friday afternoon. "Through the years I've learned that most people would rather know than not know, even if the news is bad, and especially before a weekend," she said.

The news was bad. I had breast cancer.

She tried to give me more information, but the details wouldn't penetrate at that moment. I could not absorb anything beyond "You have cancer. You will become educated." My mouth went dry.

"I can call in an order for some sleeping pills if you want."

I couldn't think. Before hanging up, I said, "Thank you."

Not thank you for the offer of pills. To that I said, "No thank you." Thank you for calling? Thank you for giving me some of the worst news I have ever gotten? I have no idea what I was thanking her for. It just came out of my mouth when nothing else would. Oh, how utterly Canadian.

That night, at my parents' house for our weekly Shabbat dinner, both my mother and father once again offered me sleeping pills. By that point we all needed them. I have no doubt that had my mother served sedatives instead of the meal she had prepared, only the children would have complained.

Over the next week, as we began telling our inner circle our horrible news, the offers of booze, drugs and medication multiplied like mushrooms (although, come to think of it, that was one thing no one offered).

"I have some OxyContin left over from my C-section. It might help."

"Would you like to try some Ativan sublingual? They're nice. It's a real easy buzz and you don't even have to swallow."

"I can offer you some of my airplane Xanax."

"Can you take codeine? I know some people are sensitive to it, but I love the way it just knocks me out cold."

"I have something they gave me when I dislocated my shoulder. I'm not sure what it is, but once you swallow you won't care."

Whether or not they had drugs to share, everybody who heard the news of my diagnosis encouraged me to drink. "It's good for what ails ya," they said. If only that were true. One friend was kind enough to deliver to my home some medical-grade marijuana. I found it in my mailbox. It made me feel nostalgic, as this very friend had been instrumental in my youthful corruption.

I had cancer, and the clear message was that I was entitled to self-medicate. But for some reason I still couldn't make the leap to prescription meds. I didn't want to go there—I think they made it all seem too real. Taking these would have meant admitting that I was not in control. It would have screamed disaster as surely as an empty jar of mayonnaise in Grammy's fridge. It is unclear to me who I was trying to fool. I hadn't been able to eat or sleep in weeks because all I could think about was having cancer.

Two weeks after my diagnosis, in the week preceding my surgery, my two younger sons came down with the chicken pox. Our friend Adrienne, always up for a mission of mercy, was beckoned to do a drugstore run late one night for calamine lotion, oatmeal bath, antihistamines, and anything else that would ease the boys' suffering and whining. I felt like Job, doing a bad impression of a parent. I tried to be comforting, but was anxious and exhausted, and the last thing I could cope with was two sick, needy children. Unfortunately, at that moment, that was precisely what I had.

Adrienne arrived, laden with just about everything she could find at the pharmacy. Into my hand she put a pill bottle with her own name on it, and the name of a friend I was about to meet, Ativan.

"Take it," she said, with enough force and conviction that I finally did.

That night, I slept. (And dreamed about sandwiches.)

4

Keep on Truckin'

WHEN MY MAMMOGRAM first showed something suspicious, I felt like I had been hit by a
truck. Afflicted by a paralysis I have known
only in dreams, when my capacity to respond to impending danger is curtailed by the reality that I am actually
asleep and I can't run to avoid being caught, or scream to
solicit help or intervention, there I lay, flattened on the
road. Each time I tried to get off the road, another truck
knocked me down. The Mack truck carrying the biopsy,
the eighteen-wheeler with the cancer diagnosis . . .
BOOM, BOOM! So stunned was I by my first vehicular
encounter, the pickup truck carrying the offending

mammogram, that I didn't even hear or see the others coming. It occurred to me that if I could just anticipate what the next truck would be carrying and when it would come, I could maybe get out of the way. To do so, I needed to think. I needed to process everything, all the time.

Naturally, a great deal of my mental energy was taken up with thoughts about my three sons. Tommy and I needed to tell our boys what was going on before my surgery—but how? What information would satisfy the curiosity of thirteen-year-old Micah without frightening Amit and Safi, who were only nine and seven? How much was enough information for them to process? How much was too much? We thought, we discussed, we plotted.

We decided on a strategy that allowed me some leeway to be wimpy in accordance with my emotionally fragile state. As it happened, my friend Maureen called and asked if I wanted to join her at a film festival screening of the new Leonard Cohen documentary. I can't claim to be a fan—Cohen is not a bad poet, but he's a terrible singer and I don't understand the virtual saint status he seems to have achieved among a certain demographic. Nonetheless, when I weighed my options—stay home and tell my kids I had cancer or go and join the Cohen cult at a premiere screening—I chose the movie. The plan was that while I was out with Maureen, Tommy would tell the boys. Under normal circumstances, I would have taken the lead on something of this sort—the delivering of crappy news in a digestible format. But Tommy, being in high protect-Ruth-at-all-costs mode, was amenable to managing it on his own. He would inform them that I needed to have an operation and that they would all have to help out. They were my team. All for one, and one for all. No need to frighten them with the "C" word. What could they possibly know or understand about cancer that would be helpful to them at this stage?

A pepperoni pizza was ordered. Tommy took a deep breath and launched in.

"Mom needs to have an operation and we're all going to have to pitch in around here," Tommy said.

"What kind of operation?" asked Safi, the youngest, his mouth full of partially chewed pizza.

"Safi, please don't talk with your mouth full," Tommy said, stalling to gather his thoughts. "Well, she has a lump in her breast and it needs to come out."

"Is it cancer?" Micah asked, grabbing for another slice before popping the last bit of crust from his previous piece into his mouth.

"Will she die?" asked Amit, focusing on the cardboard box, finger pointing at the pizza, mentally calculating how much remained for each of them.

"Does she need chemo?" somebody asked between mouthfuls.

My team had been to school, watched television, and seen movies. Coincidentally, it was Terry Fox week and the boys seemed to know everything about cancer, including what chemo was.

So after this introductory talk, we decided to change the plan and be more forthcoming with information. I knew I needed to be ready for their questions, whenever they might come up. If they didn't take me by surprise, I could be honest without frightening the boys or being knocked down myself. And so I thought about it. A lot. My mind was a virtual blender working to puree every thought, anticipation and neurosis into a well-masticated, benign pulp.

More often than not, my thought process would start somewhere reasonable. For example, how would I make the children understand that when I lost all my hair it was the treatment, not the disease that was the cause? Or, how would I respond if they asked me directly if I was going to die? After all, I couldn't guarantee anything and it would be horrible if I promised them I wasn't going to die and then I did. Not to mention that in addition to remembering me as a liar, they would inevitably become the sort of children who went to birthday parties without gifts. Or they would be the ones who couldn't go on school trips because no one had signed the proper permission forms. And people would whisper behind their backs in doleful tones, "Poor boys. You know their mother died from breast cancer . . ."

It was exhausting, but I was powerless to stop these thoughts. I had, in a matter of weeks, gone from being the cool, calm, go-to person in a crisis to being someone whose thoughts would jump in nanoseconds from "What should we have for dinner?" to "How will Tommy manage to make all the arrangements for my funeral without my help?" Where the hell is Roof?

5

@#!?* Healing Circle

"DON'T FREAK OUT, but Vera wanted me to pass on the message that she wants you to come to a healing circle," Kate said to me one day.

Since news of my diagnosis had hit the streets, my friends Kate and Cathy had been acting as my shields, screening me from the overwhelming barrage of goodwill that had erupted in the neighborhood.

"What the fuck is a healing circle?" I sputtered.

"I don't have a clue, but I did tell her that you weren't feeling up to it," Kate said. "She wasn't taking no for an answer, so I said I would pass the message on."

"Out of the question," I replied, my tone so vitriolic that it surprised me. Just the thought of what a "healing circle" might constitute made my skin crawl with New Age, crystalline offense.

"Okay, I wasn't going to tell you this, but maybe you will find it amusing. Or maybe you won't, but at least it can help fuel your fire," Kate said. "Vera says that she wants to help guide you on your journey and physically surround you with love and healing."

"Christ almighty! What the fuck does she know about guiding me? She told Cathy to tell me that 'cancer is a gift.' Don't come to my fucking birthday party if that's your idea of a gift! Last time I checked, she has never had cancer! Talk about wanting to be part of the drama!"

"Okay! Don't shoot the messenger. I'll tell her you aren't interested," Kate said, almost cowering from my poisonous onslaught.

I was not angry about having cancer. I had no feelings of the unfairness of it all, nor any "why me?" self-pity. What I did feel was intense sadness, extreme grief and debilitating apprehension, and the notion of an organized gathering so others could emote in my direction was neither what I wanted nor what I needed. It wasn't about them. This was about me.

There were those who looked at me in passing with such pain and pity that it was almost comical. There were others who avoided making eye contact altogether, lacking the social skill necessary to "say the right thing." These blunders felt more human and forgivable than the insipid saccharinity of collective healing, or the inanity of expressions of the blessing in disguise that cancer would unmask for me.

Prayers were different. I am a Jew—culturally, traditionally, unambiguously Jewish. (Religion is another matter. I have issues with organized religion.) But I figured I would take whatever good karma was offered up as long as it demanded nothing of me. When my Greek Orthodox neighbor bounded out of her house and down her porch steps to embrace me and tell me she was praying for me, it was heartfelt and sincere, and her belief, though not my own, felt genuine. My black Baptist neighbor assured me each time our paths crossed that she was praying for me. My devoutly Catholic friends on the West Coast e-mailed to tell me they were offering up a nightly family prayer on my behalf. All my Jewish friends and family included me in their weekly blessings and prayers for the sick. I was grateful for the good thoughts and spiritual bolstering from so many true believers, and equally thankful that none of them ever requested my presence at their theological encounters. Only the healing circle saw the need to physically surround me with love.

My closest friends knew instinctively that next to karaoke, or open-mike hootenannies, my least favorite pastime is going around a circle to say how you feel. What circle? you may ask. Any damn circle that imposes any outpouring of emotion in a contrived forum. My friends, from the moment of my diagnosis, surrounded me with love and healing thoughts without having to make it a game of ring-around-the-rosy.

While my response to my diagnosis was virtual paralysis, my friends shifted into high gear. Kate, Cathy, Iris and Maureen called a meeting to discuss what I needed, what my family needed, and what my community could do to get us all through this battle. Kate and Cathy organized an e-mail list of all the people in my life who might be interested in my progress, and began a correspondence with them. They created a food roster from the list for months of dinners to be delivered to our house and progress reports sent out at significant junctures in my treatment. Iris took charge of grocery shopping. Each time she went to the store herself, she called to see what our household needed and delivered our requests to our door. Maureen made sure somebody picked up my two younger boys each day after school.

I wondered how I had got so lucky as to have such wonderful friends. Not just nice, but competent! They thought of everything and then they mobilized, acted and delegated. And, of course, they demanded nothing of me in return.

When surgery was only days away, it was collectively decided that what I needed more than anything—more than consumer commodities and technological aids, more than advice or assistance, and certainly more than a healing circle—was to be distracted. What I needed was a drunken night out with good friends, good food, and foul language. What I needed was a swearing circle.

We discussed the venue and the guest list.

"Can we keep it small and close to home?" I asked. "The boys have chicken pox, so I don't want to go too far in case they need us. Also, I really don't want to deal with too many people."

"Whatever works for you," they replied. "It's your party."

We agreed to a small neighborhood restaurant within walking distance of all our houses on the Saturday night before my impending surgery. Six couples: Tommy and me, Kate and Grant, Cathy and Martin, Iris and Mike, Dave and Maureen, and Ian and Loren. All guests certain to be up to the task of a harmless bit of debauchery.

On the Sunday morning after our soiree, through bleary eyes I check my e-mail. Opening an attachment labeled

"Ruth and Tommy's @#!?* Healing Circle," I slowly examine the text and photographs. The message reads:

> Hi everyone, here's some moments from a wonderful evening celebrating life, love and laughter (not to mention the effects of beer, red wine, kirsch and grappa . . . ugh!) Our thoughts and prayers are together and strong for a swift recovery for Ruth and support for Ruth, Tommy and the boys in the weeks and months ahead. If attitude, humor, strength of spirit, and the love and support of friends and family count for anything, they are well on their way.
>
> We look forward to many more good times together . . . Thanks for a great night!
>
> Love, Cathy

This note is the first confirmation I have that the previous night has been special for others as well. In my recollection the evening has the intensity of events I remember from my teenage years. All emotion and abandon floating on the surface of empiricism, nerve endings exposed and anticipating, having the peculiar effect of heightening the good, the bad, the happy, the sad. Each joke an event, every sleight a happening. An entire life's experience lived in a single day, a night, an hour, a minute, a smile, a kiss. Everything happening now and now and now. No yesterday, no tomorrow, only now.

There are sixty-six photographs. I view them quickly as a slide show. A dinner party. Twelve friends sit around a large table that occupies much of the floor space of a restaurant. In the background of some of the pictures there are other people enjoying a night out, but the group in the foreground is getting progressively more boisterous. The increasingly manic volume is almost perceptible in the photos. The table gradually becomes covered with wine and beer bottles. The friends change positions around the table to converse with different people over the course of the evening. The first twenty pictures divulge nothing extraordinary. No one person features any more prominently than another. No special occasion is readily discernible.

I go back and view each photograph slowly, carefully. I pretend I was not there so I can try to see things more objectively. Are the people in the pictures happy or sad? They appear to be having a wonderful time, but in some of the pictures they seem engrossed in serious conversation, and in others they have tears in their eyes. What appeared to start out as an ordinary dinner party has taken a turn by the twenty-seventh photo. That one is of Tommy and me. In it I am both laughing and crying while he proudly displays my low-cut bodice for the camera.

This is a farewell party. We are bidding adieu to my right breast, and with it my cleavage. A single breast—the visual equivalent of the sound of one hand clapping.

Photo 35: Loren and Iris sharing a highly animated joke. They are enjoying themselves. They are not talking about cancer. Photo 41: Cathy and Dave posing goofily. It is not for my benefit, not for my healing. Photo 48: Grant, Ian and Mike mugging for the camera. Boys having fun. Photo 51: Me talking to Grant and Ian as I choke back tears. I recall that Grant gently held my hand for a moment, as if to say, without words, that we had his support.

Ian, trying to be serious for a moment, utters, "There is one thing I've always liked about you, Ruth."

"I hope it's not my tits," I reply, shattering his attempt at sincere sentiment.

Photos 54, 55 and 56: Group shots with Tommy and me in the front, and our friends in a semicircle behind us. I see the pose as an apt metaphor for the bittersweet nature of the gathering. Our friends may have our backs, but what we face is unknown.

As part of the bon voyage that unfolds with the help of a great deal of alcohol, everybody's décolletage—not just mine—is photographed for posterity. And so, photo number 46 shows Martin and Tommy exposing their hairy chests. Of all my male friends Martin is among the top three least likely to get carried away and take his shirt off at a restaurant, let alone allow himself to be photographed in what teeters on the edge of a compromising manner. And yet, there they are, Tommy and Martin, naked from the waist up, laughing, reveling in the moment.

This disease can't kill the good times. This disease can't steal the love. This fucking disease can't break my true healing circle.

6

Costume Party Confidence

DOCTOR H, THE SURGEON to whom I had been referred, held her clinics at one hospital, and did her operating at another. We didn't know this. Tommy, my mother and I were on time for my appointment, but at the wrong hospital. So, by the time we got to the right hospital we were late.

Being late, we had to wait, which gave us plenty of time to take in our surroundings and face some of the realities they implied. It was our first visit to the cancer centre. Everybody there, apart from the staff, either had cancer or was accompanying someone with cancer. We were no different.

None of us were complete strangers to this environment. Eighteen years earlier, we had all spent time at the
hospital with my brother during his treatment. Tommy
and I wrote all the thank-you notes for our wedding gifts
sitting in a hospital room while an IV dripped chemotherapy drugs into David's vein. That building had since
been demolished; the hospital had moved to a new location.

We tried to make conversation to pass the time. We
made eye contact with one another, so as not to see the
other patients in their cancer costumes, their bald heads,
their crooked wigs, their pale skin, their sunken eyes.
We talked about the children, and the arrangements we
had made for their care that afternoon. Who would pick
Amit and Safi up from school? Did Micah know whose
house to go to? Who would feed them dinner if we were
running late? We did not talk about the coming days or
weeks. We talked only of now and today, because although
we didn't say it, we knew that we could plan nothing
beyond the appointment for which we were waiting. The
scene had a surreal, soft-focus feel to it, as if a fog were
engulfing me. I felt a numbness, a disconnect.

Once the waiting room was empty of all the other
cancer patients, all the other family members and friends
and caregivers, we were called into the examining room.
I was ushered behind a curtain and asked to strip from
the waist up and put on a hospital gown. Emerging, I sat

between Tommy and my mother as I waited for the doctor to arrive. They put their arms around me because it was cold and I was shivering.

Dr. H came in and introduced herself. She was young and lovely and soft-spoken. Behind the quickly drawn curtain she examined my breasts and my armpits. I still can't believe that I hadn't previously noticed the large mass in my right breast. When she massaged it, it felt like an unripe apricot under my flesh. When I thought about it, I imagined a gray lump, the color of dry river rocks, hard and lifeless.

I slipped the hospital gown back over my shoulders and reclaimed the seat between Tommy and my mother. They each held one of my cold hands.

"Picture your breast from three differing perspectives," the doctor said. "If you were to look at the breast head-on in two dimensions, like the face of a clock, it is apparent from the ultrasound and mammogram reports that there are cancer cells from 10 o'clock to 2 o'clock."

One third of the pie was diseased. The protective numbness I had been affecting began to dissipate.

Then, the doctor used a cartographic image to show that the cancer covered the surface of my personal map longitudinally from collarbone to nipple. I was starting to see.

"Now," she continued, "imagine the breast in three dimensions: a small hill, a gumdrop, or half a grapefruit. According to the biopsy results, there are cancer cells in the bottom two-thirds of your three-dimensional breast."

A Halloween candy corn in which the orange and yellow portions were poisoned, and only the white tip was safe to eat.

Despite my lack of medical training, and my preconception that a lumpectomy would be recommended, with razor sharp, cutting acuity I knew before I even asked the question what I would be told. My throat felt tight and dry. With a quiver in my voice and an overwhelming sense of dread, I asked, "Are you suggesting an aggressive surgical approach?"

I think we all started crying before we even heard the answer. I know I did. With all the agonizing and processing I had been doing since the initial discovery of the lump, in my mind mastectomy had never been part of the equation. I thought it might be presented as an option, but I knew the current trend was toward breast preservation. I never imagined that having my entire breast removed would be my only choice. No wavering or exploration of creative solutions to a difficult problem. Just gut-wrenching anguish, as we felt the reality slice deeply.

I cannot equate the pain and grief I felt at that instant with anything I had ever experienced before. When I think about it now, it still makes my stomach hurt and my chest feel tight. And if I don't steel myself against my own reflexes, it still makes me cry. The intensity of those weeks and days, that moment, is beyond my ability to convey. I can recall no other time when I cried so hard and so long. I am amazed that grief and sorrow can ever be named. The capacity both to feel the pain and to communicate its depth was unfathomable to me.

I tried to tell myself that it was just a breast, not a limb. I wasn't losing an arm, or a leg, or a vital organ. I would still have all my faculties and senses intact. But this didn't help. It might be just a breast, but it was *mine*. Until now, it had been good to me. Even after three pregnancies and breastfeeding, it, or they, were still two of my best physical assets. Good shape, nice size, and terrific cleavage. So what if time and gravity had left their mark? I wore my stretch marks like a badge of honor. Now, I felt deeply betrayed.

It had been three weeks since my mammogram. It had been two weeks since my biopsy. It had been one week since my diagnosis. It would be ten days before they cut off my breast. It would be a lifetime.

—

When Amit, my middle son, was about four years old, he wanted to be Superman for Halloween. Though the stores were full of commercial interpretations, I have always believed in homemade costumes. Putting a costume together using wit, ingenuity, and whatever I could find around the house tapped into a specific type of creativity, the sort that allowed me to believe that anything was possible. As my mother and father had when I was a child, I felt it was part of my parental contract to make costumes for my children.

We found a pair of royal blue polo pajamas with green cuffs on the wrists and ankles, which we had to persuade him to wear with underpants underneath. On top of the pajamas, he wore a pair of red, jersey-knit shorts, a little too small, so they tugged a bit at the legs of the pajamas. Out of construction paper, Tommy fashioned a Superman *S* symbol that we stuck on the front of his shirt with Scotch tape. A purple satin cape was salvaged from some previous costume, and the metamorphosis was complete. Before leaving the house, Amit stopped in front of the full-length mirror by the front door and examined himself, hands on hips, with intensity. He raised his right hand to his head, and with careful, deliberate strokes, used the flat of his hand to slick his hair to the side. Returning both hands to rest on his hips, he declared with single-minded certainty, "I look exactly like him!"

When my brother David was a similar age, we went on a family outing to a spectacular magic show. It took place in a big, old theater with a gilt-framed stage flanked by heavy, red velvet curtains. The production was glitzy and theatrical. There were drum rolls, sequins, music, top hats, capes, and the most convincing, and somewhat gory, cutting in half of a woman that I have ever seen. My brother Simon and I were duly impressed, but David was enraptured. As soon as we left the theater, David was magic. Not a magician. *Magic*.

Although David could perform no tricks, no sleight of hand, no feats to amaze an audience, he was convinced of his own powers. He had all the moves and the music down pat. He would sing the tune from the show and wave his little hands around in all the appropriately magical ways. When he reached the crescendo, he would stretch his arms straight out in front, chest level, palms up, and sing "Ta-da!" and then part his arms to his sides. Nothing actually happened, but as his audience we obliged by clapping and cheering. He thought he was terrific.

One day, some older cousins and I challenged him to prove his wizardry by flying off a top bunk bed. We chanted, "Fly Magic Davey! Fly!" And he would have followed through had my auntie Riva not come in just as David was about to throw himself into free fall from a not-insignificant height. The severity of the reprimand we older children received for putting him up to such a dangerous and ridiculous stunt made him question his powers. He realized he might not actually be able to fly, ergo, he might not actually be magic. But until that moment, he was.

On the day of my surgery, I feel myself longing for the kind of confidence possessed by a boy who could be

RUTH RAKOFF

transformed into The Man of Steel by pj's and a cape.
I long to think I can embody magic and believe I can fly.
As the hospital staff walk me down the hall into the operating room, I weep. I have no costume or special powers
to shield me from my grief or my fear. I can only yearn for
the anesthetic to remove me from reality.

"Please, do it fast. Sedate me quickly," I beg as I lie
down on the cold metal table. "Please."

"This girl should have been given some Ativan," I hear
the OR nurse say as the anesthetist mercifully stabs me
with an IV needle and lets the drugs release me.

Drifting between post-anesthetic sleep and consciousness I imagine seeing an elf-like man dressed all in white.
His crisp white trousers and bright white T-shirt fit snuggly
on his small muscular frame. He has a pointy beard, a
sculpted mustache, and an almost completely shaved head.
There is a long spiky finial through a piercing in the top of
his ear. The small man lifts the covers off my body and
peeks underneath my hospital gown, exposing a thick
dressing on my chest. I don't understand why this member
of some drug-induced incarnation of the lollipop guild is
holding up a clear rubber ball filled with pinkish fluid
attached to a tube coming out of my rib cage. He is trying
to explain something to me but I can't hear him. Overcome by a sense of panic, but unable to move, I fall back

asleep. (It is not until my next hospital stay, about eight months later, that I realize that this hallucination was in fact the charming and competent post-operative nurse, who bears far less resemblance to any resident of Oz than I had imagined in my anesthetic delirium.)

When I wake again, Micah is standing next to my bed.

"Hi, Mama," he says, handing me a Three Musketeers chocolate bar. "I know you like this kind."

"Hi, Muki. Thanks. Did you come from school?" I ask as lucidly as I can manage. I remember how frightened I had felt as a child visiting my father in hospital after he underwent gallbladder surgery—he had barely looked or sounded like himself. I don't want Micah to be frightened.

"Uh-huh."

"You must be hungry," I say, giving him back the candy.

"I brought it for you," he says, taking it from me reluctantly.

"I know. That was very thoughtful of you. I'll be home tomorrow," I say, already having exhausted my capacity for conversation.

After I spend one night in hospital, the discharge planner sends me home, confident that my living situation provides me with a sufficient support system. I am overwhelmingly grateful for my life and my en suite bathroom. The home-care nurse comes every day to change my dressing and check the drain inserted at the base of my incision to collect lymphatic fluid. She assures me that everything is normal and that the drain should be able to be removed within a week or so. Normal? NORMAL? Oh, *new* normal. I close my eyes and turn my head to the side while she works just below my neck. I try to be brave and hold back my tears, but each time she visits and uncovers what I know to be my disfigured chest, I choke. The seemingly endless floodgates open, but my eyes remain tightly shut.

When the drain is removed and my wound begins to heal, I cry as I shower, still keeping my eyes closed. I touch my chest and wonder why it feels like a hollowed-out pumpkin, rather than flat like a board. (They used to tease me at school, singing "Flatsy, flatsy, Ruth's flat and that's that"—but I showed them, in good time sprouting a glorious set of D-cups.) Now I am too terrified to look. I do not want to see what I know will only deepen my sadness, my sense of profound loss. I wrap myself in a towel and dress myself with my head tilted back and my eyes looking up. I notice that the ceiling needs painting.

Sometimes the towel accidentally slips a bit, and I catch a glimpse. Where my breast used to be is a concave emptiness that starts just below my collarbone. A few times, I even try to peek beneath the towel, but I am not brave enough to look fully at my mutilated body.

—

At my post-op appointment with Dr. H, about two weeks following surgery, I turn my head away and close my eyes while she examines me.

"You haven't looked yet," she says without a hint of judgment.

"No," I reply, choking back the tumor-sized lump in my throat. "I don't have the courage."

"Let me help," she says, taking my hand in hers.

I look down at my chest and open my eyes, only to have them fill with tears that cloud my vision. The amputation is as horrible as my worst imaginings. She tells me I am brave, and I am reminded of a certain truth: bravery implies choice. Having a mastectomy had not been my choice, but it is my reality.

Like a child, I need a costume to change my reality. There is no tune, or spell, or incantation to provide me with magic. No satin cape can confer special powers. My only secret power is an invisible tit. What I need is soft and pink and made of silicone: a bionic boob, a mighty mammary.

My friend Claudia, responding to my paralysis, does all the research and asks all the questions, then provides me with a written report when she visits me after my operation: the ins and outs of being fitted with a prosthetic breast, including whom to call, where to go, and even the fact I need to bring a fitted top with me when I consult with the mastectomy fitter. I need to wait for my surgical wounds to heal before making arrangements to be fitted.

My mother takes me to the appointment. A middle-aged woman with many years of experience, the fitter, Karen, is matter-of-fact and straightforward without being harsh or abrasive. She helps make a potentially horrifying situation less jarring with her gentle professionalism and her seen-it-all attitude. As I strip down to my waist, my mother chooses not to comment on the jewel in my navel, which she is seeing for the first time. (Her life-long argument against the barbarism of piercing must seem lame and entirely beside the point in contrast to my newly mutilated body.) We leave the shop with one asymmetrical right silicone breast prosthesis in a form-fitting box, a mastectomy bra and two triangular pieces of fabric—pockets to be sewn into bras I already own, to hold my new prosthesis in place. My mother and I agree to go shopping together for something more fun sometime soon.

A few days later, dressing for a friend's party, I tuck my new prosthesis into the pocket my mother has sewn into my red lace bra. She has once again fulfilled her long-standing parental contract. My costume masks the anguish I still feel. But I can believe, if only for a time, that I am whole enough to meet the world with my eyes open.

7

Midnight Normal

AFTER ALMOST FOUR YEARS living in Israel, in the autumn of 1989 Tommy and I decided it was time to return home. Seizing the opportunity presented by leaving one life and embarking on another we took a roundabout route from the Middle East to Canada. Seven months meandering through the Far East proved to be an interesting and exciting transition between life chapters.

During our travels in India we took a detour between Calcutta and Lucknow to stop in a place called Bodhgaya. It is told that, under a banyan tree in Bodhgaya, Siddhartha attained enlightenment, and so it has become one of the four main pilgrimage centers for Buddhists from around the world. The town is filled with Buddhist temples, monasteries and gardens for prayer and contemplation. Our plan was to stay in one of the guest houses attached to a monastery, but they were all full of westerners who either had become Buddhists or were attending one of the various meditation retreats being offered in town. The only other choice for accommodation was the "tourist bungalow"—not a bungalow at all, but a crappy government-run lodge with the neglected air of a slightly dotty relative best not talked about.

Usually, particularly while traveling, I don't sleep well. Tommy, on the other hand, can sleep anywhere. That night, though, I slept soundly while Tommy was awakened by a rustling sound in our dismal room. He climbed out from under the mosquito net and followed the sound to the garbage pail, where he discovered a large rat. Startled, he grabbed the nearest thing at hand, the guest-room thermos, and dropped it into the garbage pail. Panic-stricken by the rat's ensuing screams, Tommy picked up the pail and threw the contents—rat, thermos, and all—over the third floor balcony and into the adjacent field. Returning to bed, he woke me up to tell me of his midnight murder. The buzzing of mosquitoes kept me up the rest of the night while Tommy tossed and turned with a guilt-ridden conscience. Not only had he killed a rat, but he had also sent the hotel's thermos plummeting to its demise. The following day when we checked out, we told the desk clerk about the rat (leaving out the part about throwing stuff off the balcony). With a big, beautiful smile he answered, "And my baksheesh?" Apparently, rats cost extra.

I can say with absolute certainty that I was diagnosed with cancer on September 9, 2005. I can recall with somewhat less precision that at about the same time our kitchen became inhabited by a mouse. It wasn't the first time we had reluctantly hosted rodents in our home. In the past we had set up buffet stations of what we referred to as "poison mouse medicine," because our children were taught never to touch medicine. Apparently, mice don't know they shouldn't touch "poison mouse medicine" and on each occasion they swiftly disappeared.

This mouse was different. No matter what type of bait or trap Tommy put out, we would wake each morning to find conclusive evidence that our tenant had not been evicted. Tommy became obsessed with killing the mouse, speaking about it incessantly. He got opinions from all our friends and neighbors about the best poisons, the most effective traps, the tastiest baits. He spent a small fortune at various hardware stores and specialty extermination shops on potions, concoctions, and paraphernalia guaranteed to rid us of our problem. This mouse cost extra. Come hell or high water, Tommy was going to get that mouse.

One morning, while I lay in bed in a semiconscious, post-Ativan state, I heard unusual activity from down in the kitchen. (Given that we have three sons who at the time ranged in age from seven to thirteen, sounds of unusual activity could have meant just about anything.) Tommy had gone down to the kitchen to make some coffee when he heard rustling in the pantry. Consumed by fantasies of killing the mouse, he was in unusually quick-thinking mode. (I must take a moment to qualify that statement. Tommy is exceptionally smart. He is one of those people who has always gotten straight As and won all the academic prizes there are to be won. He is a brilliant musician and all-around creative thinker. But he does not think or do things quickly. Slow and meticulous is his M.O.)

Hearing the mouse in the pantry, he grabbed the giant recycling bin we keep under the counter. He dumped the newspapers and bottles on the floor and, using the pull-out sprayer from the sink, filled the bin with water. Slowly, quietly, carefully, he pushed the tub toward the pantry. He stopped and listened. The little demon was still in there. He could hear its tiny teeth chomping on cellophane. Gingerly, he opened the pantry door—and saw his nemesis dash behind a bag of couscous. He had the mouse cornered.

First, Tommy shoved hard against all the bags and boxes of food to be certain the critter was trapped. Then, with both of his massive arms, he reached into the shelf and pulled the entire contents surrounding the mouse toward himself and into the bin of water. He had successfully drowned the mouse—along with a large quantity of dry goods. No matter, the warrior had vanquished his enemy.

Tommy came running up the stairs and announced with great excitement that he had done the deed. If cats could talk and tell of their conquests they would probably sound very much like Tommy did that morning, relating the tale of how he had entrapped that tiny beast. I swear I heard him use the expression *suffering succotash*.

Later, when he was sure that sufficient time had passed that the pest would be asphyxiated, Tommy went to clean up. One by one he removed the soggy food products from the bin of water and disposed of them. But when he was done, it was clear that there was no tiny carcass awaiting an unceremonious burial. Once again, the mouse had eluded him. The air was rife with humiliation and defeat, and to top it off, there was no Raisin Bran for breakfast.

———

During my post-mastectomy recovery, Tommy was left to take care of all the family organization, make sure there were people around to care for me and still continue to work full time. Naturally, rationally, there was no time for mouse hunting. But I was not thinking naturally or rationally. I was thinking self-referentially, through a scrim of trepidation and discomfort. When it crossed my mind that I hadn't heard about the mouse for a while, I feared that there might be a correlation between Tommy giving up on his battle with the mouse and his giving up on my battle with cancer. And since I needed him with me for the long haul, I needed to ask him about the mouse.

Tommy reported that while I had been up in bed not venturing into the kitchen, the mouse had been digging in, getting bolder, and consuming ever more pasta. We needed reinforcements, in so many ways.

When my brother David came from New York about a week after my surgery to help take care of the boys and me, he inadvertently got conscripted into war with the rodent during his three-week stay. Late one night, after giving me my medications, emptying my surgical drains, propping my arms up with the requisite number of pillows of precisely the right texture, supporting my neck with pillows of a different texture, removing the pea from beneath my mattress, and generally settling me into bed, Tommy and David went down to the kitchen for a snack.

Late-night snacking has always been one of my family's great, shared pleasures. I think it also reminded them of being teenagers, coming home at all hours, raiding my mother's refrigerator, with no concern for calories, cholesterol, or what someone else might have planned for the available delicacies. (As an adolescent David once polished off an entire leg of lamb intended for the next day's dinner, one small slice at a time.) Standing in a dark kitchen, but for the light of the open fridge door, like locusts Tommy and David could systematically clear the shelves of everything save a few jars of jam and jelly.

The heaviness of our current burden made the need for nocturnal snacking more poignant. The void left by my inability to eat or take pleasure in food was cavernous and unfamiliar to all of us. Everyone else felt the need to dig in with extra gusto. So off they went to enjoy a simple midnight snack and forget, if only for a moment, that we had entered a different dimension. A new normal where people took care of me instead of me taking care of them. A parallel universe where I lay in bed, instead of standing by the fridge door sharing a snack with the boys.

When Tommy turned on the kitchen light, the mouse boldly scurried across the floor and hopped up into the pantry through a slightly gaping door. Immediately Tommy went into commando mode and pushed David up against the pantry doors.

"What the hell . . ." David screeched, startled by Tommy's aggressiveness.

"Just hold the doors closed so the bloody mouse doesn't escape!" Tommy barked.

"No way," said David, attempting to abandon his post. "I don't want any part of this." With the force of a hard-core military leader, Tommy gave the order: "Don't even think about moving!"

Meanwhile, he assembled his arsenal. At the base of the pantry, he created a patchwork of aluminum foil baking pans filled with water.

David, feeling completely cowed by Tommy's crazed behavior said, "What the fuck are you doing?"

Tommy excitedly explained, "When the mouse leaves the pantry it will land in the water. It might not be enough to drown it, but I hope to at least slow it down enough to get at it."

Armed with a carving knife like the proverbial farmer's wife, Tommy opened the pantry. Catching sight of a tail, he began poking around with the knife, coaxing the mouse toward the opening. It is unclear if David's high-pitched shrieking helped or hindered the operation, but as planned, the mouse was left with only one choice. Kamikaze-style, it dove head first into the foil pool and tried valiantly to swim toward the edge. Before the mouse could get to safety, Tommy brought the knife down.

At that point, David went AWOL and came running up the stairs. Breathlessly, he sat down, whimpering, on my bed. "Ruthie, are you up?"

"Ya, I'm up. What the hell is going on down there?" I asked.

"The kitchen is a war zone," he muttered. "Your husband is like a man possessed."

We sat and listened to the noises coming from down below. David gagged on his own words: "He chopped the mouse in half and blood splattered everywhere. I'll never sleep again."

We lay on my bed in the dark, like we had as children when he would come to my room after a nightmare. Scarier things than the bedtime imaginings of a small child haunted our world now, so we focused on the horror of the victimized mouse, and waited.

As though to the darkness of a confessional, Tommy came upstairs and declared, "I didn't actually kill the mouse. It must have died of shock when the knife chopped off its tail."

He lay down on the bed next to David and opened a bag of chips he had salvaged from the battlefield wreckage of the kitchen. As they had done so many times before, the two of them found solace in the salty, greasy crunch of midnight normal.

8

Cancer Present

EIGHTEEN YEARS AGO, when my brother was diagnosed with Hodgkin's disease at age twenty-two, my parents bought him a beautiful, three-quarter length, rich pebbled leather jacket. It was one of those "timeless classic" pieces of expensive clothing, bought with either conscious or subconscious aspirations that he would be around to wear it for a very long time. It fit him beautifully and provoked compliments on a regular basis from both friends and strangers. He looked stylish and groomed no matter what was going on beneath the layer of the coat. "Thank you," my brother would reply shyly to people he didn't know, who had no idea what he was going through. To people he did know he would say "Thanks, it's my cancer present," more cheerily than he possibly could have felt.

Each time I heard him say "cancer present," something in me would bristle. I didn't have the life experience at twenty-four to understand any of the reasons why a cancer present was important. I didn't understand the profound impotence my parents must have felt in their inability to provide a real solution to the problem, genuine comfort, a guarantee, a cure. I didn't understand that buying an expensive gift was an act of defiance. I didn't understand that they desperately needed to do something, anything, to make a difference, to help. My lack of understanding even extended to a faint hope that my parents' cancer generosity might have a trickle-down effect and I too might score a cool gift. A "my brother has cancer" consolation prize akin to what is given to children who don't win at sporting events: satin ribbons embossed in gold lettering with the word *Participant*.

When I was diagnosed with cancer and my world came crashing down around me, we grasped at anything that might make it better. By "we," I mean me, my family and my friends. By "it," I mean the whole daunting package that a cancer diagnosis brings. People who cared for me arranged everything from outings to distract me, flowers to brighten up my home, medication to sedate me, food to nourish me, treats to spoil me, and visitors to both cheer and console me—a plethora of all.

My friends determined that for my bedroom to be a good place to convalesce it needed some tweaking. A new bedside lamp, a headboard for comfortable reclining, new pillows for my bed, chair cushions for my reading chair, a special armchair-type bed rest, new phones with a built-in intercom for easy communication throughout the house, comfortable pajamas, and a soft bathrobe with a wide, shawl collar to help camouflage what would be my missing breast.

They shopped with me and without me. My preoccupation left me incapable of making any decisions, so they made them for me. A soft, red cushion with polka dots and a pale green seat pad for the wicker chair by the window, pink and white striped cotton pj's and the fluffiest of fluffy pale blue robes all awaited my post-operative return from hospital. A specialty garment researched by Kate on the Internet to be worn after a mastectomy was brought to me in a pretty pink box I was unable to bring myself to open until I absolutely had to, the delicacy of its packaging and lace neckline cold comfort for the harsh truth it represented. A hot pink faux-suede backrest pillow and a faux rabbit-fur bed throw, both perfect matches for my soon-to-be faux bosom. I had everything—including cancer.

Still, out of some perverse interpretation of entitlement, it occurred to me that I should buy myself a cancer present, something lavish and extravagant that I would never consider under normal circumstances. I am someone who takes great pride in my ability to feed and clothe my family frugally with discount brands and flyer specials. When purchasing produce, I religiously stick to my ninety-nine-cent rule—if it's more than ninety-nine cents a pound, I don't buy it. That's not to say that I don't succumb to the occasional sacrilegious indulgence, but my idea of a splurge is buying berries in the dead of winter, or an entire case of local cherries in season. A fine-tip pen, a pair of sparkly flip-flops, a serving platter—any of these things might, under normal circumstances, appeal to my sense of want, not need—my implicit understanding of the definition of a gift. But, alas, I could think of nothing great or small that I wanted.

My inability to think of a gift for myself had nothing to do with money. Money was no object. Not that we suddenly had plenty to spare—we didn't. But the bank had lots and they were happy to share it with us. Given socialized health care and a good benefits package through Tommy's employer, we didn't have to worry about the direct costs of cancer. Doctors were covered. Procedures were covered. Home-care nursing and physiotherapy—check. Medication—check. Even fake hair and artificial boob were covered by a combination of workplace insurance and government subsidy for medical devices. Some indirect costs, of course, such as my complete withdrawal from the workforce, and the hiring of someone to help clean and do laundry, were squeezing us a little. But in the grand scheme of things a few extra expenses felt like a minor inconvenience. Incurring some debt wouldn't put us in the position of worrying about losing our home, or having our car or furniture repossessed.

In the past, I would have avoided dipping into our line of credit. If we couldn't afford it, we couldn't have it. If we wanted something, we would save for it. I preferred to pay cash for things than to put them on credit. I know it sounds positively Amish and quaint. After all, everybody has debt. Everybody uses credit cards, probably even the Amish. But the notion of living beyond our means made me disproportionately uncomfortable.

Browsing in a boutique with my friend Cathy a couple of days post-diagnosis, I came across a pair of ankle socks. They were a beautiful jewel-tone red of the softest, plushest chenille-type fabric I had ever felt. I squeezed and caressed the socks on their tiny plastic hanger.

"Buy them," Cathy said, seeing the look of desire in my eyes.

"Are you crazy?" I replied in a tone best reserved for matters of genuine crisis or wails of hallelujah. "They cost thirteen dollars!" (Far in excess of the two-dollar sock rule, and even surpassing the ten-dollar T-shirt rule.)

"Ruth, you have cancer, for fuck sakes. Buy the fucking socks."

I bought the socks. With the aberrant purchase of the thirteen-dollar socks, my lifelong attitude about money and debt dissolved. My cancer diagnosis had created a shift even in my inbred attitude to debt. "It's just money," I said. And everybody knew exactly what I meant.

And yet, I still couldn't think of an appropriate cancer gift. The socks didn't fit the bill.

I used to get a perverse thrill out of watching my lapsed Catholic friend Jeanette squirm with naughty delight when, in my best imitation of a 1970s hostess with the mostest (I imagine myself in a paisley maxi dress in this role). I would pass around trays of snacks offering "Body of Christ, anyone?" No matter how many times I made the same stupid joke, it never failed to amuse us both. These few words had the capacity to make us regress to school days long past. Jeanette was instantly back being overseen by dour nuns, a Catholic schoolgirl substituting dirty words for standardized hymns under cover of cacophony, and I was the loudmouth class clown saying what others dared not even think.

When I met my medical oncologist for the first time a

few weeks after my mastectomy, he offered me chemotherapy. Not as in "would you like a martini?" but as an
additional lifesaving measure. I confess that in my mind
he was offering "Body of Christ"—an offer of a higher
order, not a smartass quip on a platter. He presented it as a
choice based on the facts. I had stage II, estrogen-positive
breast cancer, with nodular and lymphovascular involve-
ment, meaning that although I had just had my entire
breast, nipple and all, removed, as well as all the lymph
nodes in my right armpit, without chemotherapy I could
not be sure that there was no cancer left in my system.
Even with chemo, there were no guarantees, but my sta-
tistical outcomes would be better. How could I say no to
that kind of offer? In my mind, I had no choice—par for
the cancer course. I imagine that confirmed Catholics
don't refuse the host during Communion: it's just "not
done." As a confirmed cancer patient I was resigned to
kneeling down and opening wide for the toxic chemicals.

My oncologist wanted to start my chemo protocol the
following week. Grasping at straws, and desperate in
my need to control some aspect of my spiraling-out-of-
control life, I said I needed a couple of weeks to put some
things in order.

What could I possibly put in order? The big things were
so big that the little things were beyond me. I couldn't
even decide what to eat or what to wear without major

angst. I called upon a tried-and-true method of organizational genius. I made a list:

> breast
> wig
> hair

Linda had been expecting my call. Linda is not only my hairdresser, she is a friend and a member of our close-knit community. A couple of years earlier I had introduced Linda and Claudia when Claudia had been diagnosed with breast cancer. Linda had taken Claudia through her hair loss paces: cutting her hair short prior to chemo, styling the wig she bought, and feigning nonchalance when she clipped Claudia's hair close, as it released itself from her scalp in bunches a couple of weeks after starting chemo.

"I need to come see you," I said.

"Any time," she said.

"I need to get a wig before I cut my hair short so I can try to match my usual look." These were the things I could control. I was in charge.

I made two other appointments. The first was the one with the mastectomy fitter. The second was with a wig mistress whose name had been given to me by my cousin

Faye. All I had to do was make the appointments and show up. Easy peasy lemon squeezy.

After spending close to seven hundred dollars on a fake boob and fake hair, thereby crossing two things off my "to do" list, I felt awful. I had hoped taking charge of these controllable details would help me regain some sense of order, but instead I felt even more defeated. I didn't want my prosthetic breast, I wanted my real one. I didn't like the wig, I liked my real hair. The choices I had made were pseudo choices.

"Would you like to go on this luxury cruise or just stay home and flip through the brochure?"

"Would you like chocolate or vanilla, or this yummy-looking picture of ice cream?"

I tried to look forward to my haircut, to see it as an opportunity. Here was a chance I might never have gotten on my own. I could cut my hair short and see how it looked. If I hated it, it didn't really matter, because it would all fall out in a few weeks. If I liked it, all the better. My glass was half full.

Cathy came with me to Linda's. We were going to make a day of it. A haircut, lunch, some shopping—girl time we almost never get. As Linda's scissors skillfully snipped my long locks into a short stylish coiffure, I felt the optimism draining from me. With each clump of hair that fell to the floor, adding to the mound at the base of my chair, I found it harder to hang on to my fabricated delusion. I didn't really want a short haircut. I didn't really care to see what it looked like. When it was done, I felt powerless, like Samson. What I lacked in choice, I made up for in narcissism, elevating the event of my haircut to biblical stature.

So that was it, the end of my list—hair, wig, breast—all under control. *I'm ready for my close-up, Mr. DeMille*, I thought, having never felt less ready in my life.

Despite feeling overwhelmed and vanquished, I went with Cathy down to Queen Street to continue with our plan. I gazed from the car window into the storefronts in the early stages of holiday season readiness, silently calculating that by the time the holidays actually rolled around, all things being well, I should be halfway through my chemo treatments. Endless windows, displaying sweaters and coats and boots, appeared to pass before my eyes, as though I were standing still and the storefronts were on the move. Hundreds and hundreds of pairs of black and brown boots: high-heeled boots, flat-soled boots, leather boots, suede boots, boots with laces, boots with buckles, lined boots, sensible boots—all on the move.

"I need a pair of boots," I blurted out, semi-conscious that there was almost nothing I needed less than boots three days before starting chemo. Other than hospitals,

I had nowhere to go. By the time chemo ended winter would be almost over.

"Okay, then, let's go boot shopping," Cathy replied, ever accommodating to my unpredictable whims.

"I need plum-colored boots," I said, with a conviction that surprised me. Plum-colored boots would be my cancer present. Anybody could choose black boots, or brown boots, but one had to have special powers to find plum-colored boots in the sea of black and brown. *I choose plum-colored boots*, I thought. *I choose. I choose. I choose.*

"All right, let's go find you plum-colored boots," Cathy said.

At that moment, I was grateful to Cathy for sharing my conviction that there would undoubtedly be plum-colored boots for me to buy.

In and out of Queen Street shoe stores we went, energetically searching for the perfect boots. "Just looking," we said, as we quickly scanned the merchandise displayed in each store, certain that when they were there we would see them, like bright stars in the night sky, easily distinguishable from the rest.

Intermingled with the black and brown, a blue pair, an orange pair, red leather in the shape of traditional gum boots, boots with embroidered dragons . . . And then, there they were—my plum-colored boots, flat-soled, square-toed, and made of leather and suede and elasticized ribbon, that I had willed into existence. I did not check the price. Did Cinderella ask, "How much are these glass slippers?"

Along with the boots, I bought a special brush to tend the delicate suede, and some weather-proofing spray. I would take good care of my plum-colored boots. I needed them to last for many winters to come.

9

˙ When the Bough Breaks

MY MOTHER SITS reading a book in the pale green wicker chair by the long window at the top of the stairs, at the entrance to my third-floor loft bedroom. She is not good at sitting still. Even when she reads, she does so with fervor and activity, always hungry for more, always afraid of missing out. With one hand, she holds her hardcover edition—too impatient to wait for the paperback—that rests half on the arm of the chair and half on her thigh. An object at rest remains at rest. An object in motion remains in motion. She dares not rest for fear of remaining at rest. With her other hand, arm raised above her shoulder, elbow bent, she tugs at single strands of hair at the crown of her head, gently pulling strand by strand. She has always done so while reading. I do not need to look at her to know what she is doing.

In my semi-cognizance I hear the phone ring softly. Though technologically challenged, my mother has managed to quiet the tone. It's her job, her duty, to do so. She answers quickly after only one ring.

"Hello," she says quietly into the phone. "This is her mother. She is resting now."

Patiently, for the umpteenth time, she replies to the heartfelt query on the other end of the line. "She is doing all right today. We just did her exercises and now she's tired. Thank you for phoning. I'll tell her you called," she says, keeping the conversation brief. She is tired too. After all, she has been hyper-conscious during my convalescence. At least I have had the benefit of sedatives.

The doorbell rings and with my eyes closed I hear my mother hoist herself out of the creaky chair and descend the two steep flights of stairs to the main floor, her stiffened joints slowing her progress. Shortly after, I hear her returning with a faint "Oy," a stifled acknowledgment of her many trips up and down the many stairs.

"Are you okay?" I ask, opening my eyes as she enters my room. I see that she is carrying yet another beautiful, elaborate flower arrangement.

"Yes. I'm fine. Some more flowers. Rest," she says,

finding a spot for the newest arrivals between two equally spectacular bouquets on the dresser beside my bed. She pulls slightly at the blooms, separating them in their glass vase till she is satisfied by their presentation, eliminating random disorder. Controlling what she can.

My bedroom looks and smells like a greenhouse. Dozens of deliveries from florists have arrived since my return from hospital. I close my eyes and, with the smell of blossoms in my nostrils, I fall into a deep, drug-induced slumber.

I awake some time later to the sound of footfalls on the stairs. My mother leads the way, followed by one of what will be many visitors. I must have slept for a long time because she has decided that it is okay to wake me. She is the gatekeeper. She determines entry.

"All right, I'll make tea while you have a visit." With the arrival of reinforcements, the sentry can leave her post. Leaving the visitor seated by my bedside, my mother turns and heads back down the stairs, again the echo of her pace divulging her aching knees, hips, feet and back. The tintinnabulation of cups gently clinking against saucers announces my mother's return. Another trip up the many stairs from the kitchen.

"You shouldn't be climbing the stairs carrying such a heavy tray," I say impotently, knowing I cannot offer to carry it for her.

"Actually," she says breathlessly as she reaches the top step, "the exercise is good for me.

"Now, you must try and eat something," she decrees, arranging the tea tray on the bed tray next to me. She has brought toast with Vegemite, cut into fingers, in case I might be enticed to eat something salty. She has brought chocolate biscuits, no doubt from one of the many care packages that have been delivered, in case it is sweetness that I crave. There is a small bowl of deep red strawberries that have been carefully hulled and sliced in half, exposing their pink innards, fresh and strangely pungent. The smell of the berries, mixed with the lilies and roses, sends a wave of nausea through me.

My mother pours tea for me and my visitor. "Encourage her to eat something," she says to our guest.

"I'll have some of the toast," I say to make her happy. I know I will not eat it.

"I'm going to make you some soup for later," she says, heading back toward the stairs. She doubles back and ducks into the bathroom, grabbing the laundry basket. It is almost empty, but I have given up trying to tell her that she doesn't have to do laundry all the time.

Carrying the basket, she heads back downstairs. This time I hear her painful padding all the way to the basement, the creak of the ancient steps giving voice to what her body feels and her mouth suppresses. She will start the laundry. She will make some soup. She will climb back up to my bedroom and tell my visitor when it is time to go. She will once again make the descent to escort the departing friend to the front door. She is not good at sitting still.

My mother does not like to speak about her mother. Protective even beyond the grave, as though giving voice to the many sadnesses that plagued my grandmother's life might cause them to be relived, reexperienced. The topic of her own mother's life is one of the few that cracks my mother's stoic exterior, even almost half a century after my grandmother's death. My mother does not recall an unhappy childhood of deprivation or neglect. But when asked about her mother, it is the tragic details she recounts. She is who she is because of the difficulties and struggles of her early life, her mother's life, the life of the father she never knew. The fever pitch with which she lives her life betrays this. She misses nothing—symphony, opera, readings, ballet; she is at every event around town. And the nights she is home she is entertaining. She pursues FUN as though it were a mission to accomplish as only someone who has felt the sting of deprivation, of missing out, of grief, can.

I call my mother on the phone from my yellow couch to clarify some of the details of her early life. In light of our recent experiences, I believe she will answer questions she might have been reluctant to in the past.

In 1930, at the age of thirty-four, my grandmother, Betty Bahn, crossed the ocean from Latvia to South Africa in search of a better life.

"Why wasn't she married?" I ask my mother. "Thirty-four would have been old in those days."

"I don't know." The words catch in my mother's throat. The question upsets her. "Maybe they were too poor," she guesses. "What's all this about?" she wants to know.

"I'm trying to write something. I want to get it right," I say. My mother does not know that I have been writing. So far it is my private pursuit.

She followed her sister Gene, already married by arrangement and settled in South Africa, leaving her four other siblings behind, never to see them again. In those days, an escape across the ocean represented a finality we can no longer fathom. The world was much bigger then. Though not formally educated past the age of twelve, Betty spoke Yiddish, German and Russian. Upon arrival in South Africa, she also learned Afrikaans and English.

"I was so ashamed of her heavy accent and bad grammar," my mother recalls. "God, I was so foolish. I didn't realize what an accomplishment it was for her."

I do not remind my mother that as a child my brother was embarrassed by *her* foreign accent. Before the guests arrived for his fourth birthday party, my brother said to my mother, "Don't talk. You talk funny." She does not bear a grudge—he was a child. She holds herself to a higher standard.

"When we moved to Canada, she wrote to me in English. I didn't write to her in Yiddish," my mother says, still wrestling with the ghosts of guilt. "I have all of her letters."

"I'd like to see them," I say.

"I'll find them some time," she replies, reluctant to wake the dead and expose emotions that are still raw if stirred even slightly.

In 1931, Betty married a widower named Simon Shochat. They honeymooned at Muizemberg Beach with Simon's two young sons, ages five and eight. "I have pictures of all of them on honeymoon, somewhere," she says. The boys had been living since their mother's death with a kindly aunt and a nasty, abusive uncle. My mother's brief description of her brothers' time with Uncle Zalman is Dickensian, with a heavy Yiddish accent. My mother wasn't there, so the tales are hearsay. Nonetheless, she cannot forgive or forget.

"He was a real bastard," she says, preternaturally coarse. She still feels the need to protect her brothers—one long dead, the other a man in his eighties.

Uncle Zalman is the first on my mother's list of good versus evil. She has been subconsciously compiling her list since she was born. It is only in the past decade or so, however, that I became aware of, and gave name to, "the list." The good list is longer than the evil list, but once someone is on one side or the other, there is very little that can change their category. On the good list is a collection of people, mostly women, who are either wonderfully energetic, competent and accomplished, or pathetic, hard-done-by and needy in a variety of permutations. Both "good" groups can easily be identified by my mother's response to the mention of their names in conversation. When the name of one of the "good" powerhouses comes up, I silently start counting in my head, "One an two an three an . . ." Inevitably, before I get very far in the count, my mother pipes in with "She's terrific!" *She* is on the list.

The unfortunate members of the good list are those in need of help and care, dominated by a sadly growing number of widows, widowers, orphans and the critically ill or disabled, or caregivers of the ill or infirm. The mention of these folk can be met with either a "she's terrific" or, more likely, "shame." Not shame in the American sense of the word—as in, an embarrassment or humiliation. Rather, "shame" in the South African sense—as in, pitiful or pathetic to the point of inspiring sympathy and empathy. My mother is impressed by the go-getters and energized by the needy.

The members of the evil list tend not to be people who

have personally wronged my mother. More often than not they have hurt or wronged people or causes my mother cares deeply about. Things that seem to put evil-doers firmly in their column are disloyalty, betrayal, greed, grandiosity, cruelty and other such sins.

The only way to go from evil to good is to suffer. One must grieve the loss of a significant loved one, or succumb to critical illness. Only then can my mother's mind remarkably eliminate any recollection of evildoing. But such a shift is rare. Her lists are like her own private religion and she is spiritual leader and devoted follower rolled into one fervently faithful being.

Shortly after they wed, Betty and Simon Shochat moved from one small town, Montague, to Worcester, another small town. Betty raised the boys and worked alongside her husband in the general store he had purchased with capital assistance from a local philanthropist (good list). In 1936, my grandmother delivered my mother, Gina, by pre-term caesarian section at a big-city hospital in Cape-town. When I was pregnant with my first child, I began to question my mother about her own pregnancies, and my grandmother's pregnancy. "I don't really remember," my mother said, reluctant to divulge any information. Her superstition about not buying anything for my unborn child struck me as primitive and odd for such a woman as no-nonsense, pragmatic, and pathologically organized as my mother. It wasn't until after the birth of my first son, and only when speaking of the tragic, full-term stillbirth of a friend's baby, that I learned that my grandmother herself had suffered three full-term stillbirths before she had my mother. It wasn't that it was a secret, just that it was too painful for my mother to recall how much her mother had endured. Only then did I understand her reluctance to prepare until Micah was safely among us.

After my mother was born, her father purchased the property adjacent to the store and built a house for his family. It was a two-story house, with a balcony that ran the length of it at the back, and a smaller balcony at the front.

"It was a nice balcony," she recalls. "There was a bird-cage in the back. I wonder what ever happened to those canaries . . . I guess they died as well."

She digresses. "I had a dog, you remember, named Gibor." Gibor, the Hebrew word for "brave." "When your father and I moved to Canada in 1961, Gibor stayed with my mother in South Africa. She wrote me in a letter that Gibor had died. I cried and cried," she says sheepishly, embarrassed at having wept for her dog. But it is another loss associated with her mother, her connection to South Africa, her childhood.

"The staircase in the house had a wonderful wooden banister that all the children used to slide down."

But she doesn't indulge long in this nostalgic interlude, instead returning to the heartbreaking chronology. "My father died shortly after we moved into the house."

"When you were three?" I ask, trying to put history in place.

"No, when I was two. They kept him in bed too long after a minor operation. It was a hernia. He died from a post-operative pulmonary embolus. That's how they did it then. It's different these days. They get patients up right away. He shouldn't have died so young," she says, barely resigned to his fate after almost seventy years.

"What happened after he died?" I ask, searching for clues and comprehension.

"What do you mean 'what happened'?" She sounds irritated, as though it's a stupid question.

"I mean what happened to your mother, and the business, and the house? Who took care of you?"

"After my father died, my mother had a sort of breakdown. She just couldn't cope." My mother's voice cracks. The answer breaks her heart. "He died without a will. So my mother had to go and ask the authorities—I can't remember exactly who—the court or the public something or other, for money from the estate, to live on. She was broken and so humiliated, having to ask for money. It was awful."

I'm starting to have a keener understanding of my mother's need to control. The Fates began to conspire against her early on. *Always complete a task*, I hear her saying in my childhood ears, the words echoing in my adolescent brain, my adult mind, watching her almost compulsively tidying, straightening, putting in order, leaving nothing to chance.

"My brothers were wonderful. They really took good care of me. Michael was like a father—he always made me feel very cherished. Poor Michael." Michael is on the good list, one of the ones elevated to virtual saint status. Despite glaring, obvious character flaws, one dare not even hint at anything negative about him in my mother's presence. She will not hear it. In her version of life, her brother Michael is a divine being. So, I am surprised by her next reminiscence.

"Michael was only fifteen years old when our father died. My mother couldn't manage. She had suffered too many losses. I guess she was depressed. So at fifteen, he took over the business. But you know, he had his own problems. He was a kid, and he had a gambling problem. His whole life he did. He ran the business into the ground. It went bankrupt by the time I was fourteen. We lost everything—the business, the house—everything." Time has provided only a thin filter for her sadness. It is as though it were yesterday.

"What sort of relationship did you have with your mother?" I ask, knowing pieces of the answer from conversations over time with other members of the family. But I want to hear it from her.

"I remember looking after her from a very young age," she says, confirming what I've heard. "I remember making dinner. I couldn't have been more than ten. She had nothing to look forward to. Really nothing. She had losses and rheumatic pain. When she was fifty she became diabetic. When she was sixty she suffered a stroke. At sixty-seven she died of colon cancer.

"Dad and I shouldn't have left when we did," she says, referring to my parents' emigration to Canada in 1961.

"Your mother didn't have cancer when you left, did she?" I ask.

"She didn't have a diagnosis—but who knows? I went back a year and a half later to take care of her. You were three weeks old and your brother Simon was two. I made the doctor do the caesarian as early as possible so I could go take care of my mother. Can you imagine? Three weeks post-op, traveling with a newborn and a two-year-old all the way from Montreal to South Africa."

My mother has always been a caregiver. It is what she does best. She never had any choice.

——

My mother takes me to every doctor's appointment. As is often the case, the resident enters the examining room before the doctor. With my chart tucked under his arm he casts his gaze at my mother.

"Ms. Rakoff?" he asks.

"It should be me," my mother replies with a deep sadness that catches in her throat. "Excuse me," she adds with a small cough. "I'm her mother."

She sits through one appointment after another, quietly observing. She has put her life on hold. She does not speak. She does not ask questions. My mother lets me do the talking. Her medical experience is not her calling card on these occasions. She is there as a mother. She listens to understand what will be expected of her as my caregiver. "You might want to try eating a light breakfast on chemotherapy days," Dr. C, my oncologist, suggests. "Nothing that is your favorite. If you do feel sick from the treatment, it can put you off some things forever."

"What if I don't feel like eating?" I ask.

"It's not essential to eat, but you must drink a lot, particularly after treatment," he replies.

My mother makes a mental note; I can sense it. She will not force me to eat.

"You will need to have blood work done before each treatment. After you have your blood drawn at the hematology lab you must go to the chemotherapy clinic waiting area. Let them know you're there so they can tell you when your blood results come back," the oncology nurse instructs.

"What do my blood counts need to be?" I ask, knowing my mother will listen for the answer.

Like every morning, Tommy gets up before me and prepares a cup of ginger tea that he places on my bedside table before waking the children and me. On chemo days my mother leaves her house while it is still dark, so she can pick me up on time for our early morning appointment. She drops me at the entrance to the cancer center so I do not have to walk too far. She parks the car and joins me outside the hematology lab. I watch her as she crosses the threshold of the hospital. She is small. Her boots seem too big. She carries her lunch in a small rectangular cooler bag. Her flashy silver purse hangs heavy on her shoulder. She clutches a book in one hand. She moves quickly, but with the halting gait of someone in pain. To anyone else, she must look like an old woman. She takes her glasses off the top of her head and places them on her face. She scans the waiting room for me, the shimmer of her pale blue eye shadow enhanced by the reflection off the glasses. She spots me and comes to sit with me.

We wait.

"Did you have any breakfast?" she asks.

"No, did you?" I reply.

"Yes, of course I did," she says. "It's a long day." She is not complaining, merely stating the truth.

I go to the bathroom to put an EMLA anesthetic patch on the Port-A-Cath embedded in my chest. By the time they hook me up for chemo, my skin should be numb enough to not feel the sharp stick of the needle. I peel the small patch off its foil backing and gently place it over the bump in my chest. Carefully, I press down the adhesive edges, sealing in the cream. I lay my fingers flat against the patch, pushing softly to ensure contact between skin and salve. I dread even one more needle. When I return, my mother seems twitchy, agitated.

"I'm going to get a cup of coffee," she says. "Would you like anything, maybe some tea?"

She takes the opportunity to go for a stroll to the coffee shop before the treatment begins. Once it starts, she will not leave my side.

When it takes a long time for my blood work to come back, my mother steps outside to call her office. She has cleared her schedule on chemo days, but checks in just in case. She must leave the hospital to be a doctor.

During the long hours that the poisons drip into me, I sleep. The drugs knock me out. I am not good company. My mother sits beside me and reads, pulling at the white hair at the crown of her head. I wake with a full bladder many times from the saline infusion that accompanies my chemo cocktail. My mother holds my arm and pushes my IV pole as she guides me to the bathroom. I am dizzy and lightheaded.

"Do you need me to come in with you?" she asks.

"I think I can manage."

"I'll be right outside." She waits by the heavy door, and pushes it open for me as soon as she hears the turn of the handle that signals I'm done.

At midday, she unzips her small cooler bag and removes a sandwich. She takes half a sandwich from its wrapper and carefully refolds the tinfoil over the other half. She always completes a task. She eats one half, unwraps the other half, and refolds the foil, putting it back into her bag. She will reuse it. She is phobic about waste.

"Would you like to eat something?" she asks.

"No," I reply. I cannot make conversation. She continues to read.

She stands to stretch. It is difficult for her to sit. Her back aches. She flexes her pelvis, pushing her lumbar curve against the wall. She stretches her arms above her head, holding her right wrist with her left hand, pushing up on the balls of her feet. Stretched from toe to fingertip, she does not reach the top of the IV pole.

A volunteer comes around offering coffee and cookies. My mother is shy about accepting, believing they are for the patients. She is an interloper, unentitled.

"Are you sure you won't have something, dear?" the volunteer asks. She sees my mother's fatigue. She sees my mother's age.

My mother changes her mind. "Just some coffee would be lovely. Thank you." She has been sitting now for many hours.

I accept a small cellophane package containing two plain white biscuits. When the volunteer leaves the room, I pass them to my mother.

"Don't you want them?" she asks me.

"I changed my mind," I say, knowing that she will eat them, if only to pass a moment, to create a break in the monotony.

"Do you have a hard candy?" I ask, my mouth parched from the drugs.

My mother rummages in her silver purse. "I don't have any," she laments. "Isn't that strange," she says. "I always have candies, and just when you want one I don't have any." Next chemo she will bring me six rolls of Lifesavers.

I pick up my "at home" meds from the cancer center pharmacy while she goes to retrieve the car, saving me the trek. I discuss the protocol with the pharmacist. It is different each time because none of the antinausea drugs seem to work. They give me a schedule of what to take and when. Some days I am taking more than thirty pills.

I get into the car and hand my mother the schedule. She will take care of it. She will take care of me.

Like clockwork, I begin to vomit two hours after the end of each treatment. I have eaten nothing, so all that comes up is a profuse volume of water, ginger tea and bile. I retch violently and repeatedly, making horrible, frightening, heaving sounds. I worry that my children can hear me. My mother holds my head to protect it from hitting the toilet bowl. She places one hand firmly on my forehead, and the other on my shoulder, knowing intuitively that I need to be physically stabilized. Her cool hands feel refreshing against my skin. I remember them on my feverish face as a child.

When the episode passes, I am spent. I crumple from my perch above the porcelain and lie down on the cool blue tiles of the bathroom floor. My mother wets a washcloth with tepid water and strokes it on my forehead and the back of my neck. Kneeling beside me on the hard floor, she rests my head on a stack of towels and cradles me. I am comforted by the feel of the loose skin on her arms. It is soft and malleable. I ease into it. She guides me back to my bed and helps me change into clean pajamas. She tucks me in.

By the time I am through eight rounds of chemo, my insides are raw. It hurts to swallow, and my digestive tract can absorb nothing. The water I force down in tiny, excruciating sips rushes through my body as though I have sprung a leak. It hurts my mother to see me suffer. I yearn to find the strength to put on a good face to protect my mother, my children and my spouse from my pain.

I cannot tolerate anything sweet. The drugs have done something to my taste buds and sweet tastes unbearably sour.

"If only there were something soft and savory that would slide down without touching the sides of my throat," I say.

"That's not possible," my mother says. "Your muscles must contract in order for you to swallow." She can be very literal.

My mother searches the depths of her imagination to come up with the ideal food. She prepares a cheese soufflé. It is the lightest, airiest, softest, most benign substance in the universe. She practically spoon-feeds it to me, offering me more than I can manage. I ease the food down my gullet with my tongue. I am like an infant in need of cradling and soft food.

My mother stands at the ready to catch me after each fall I suffer on this journey. She does not flinch or stumble from the burden. It is her mission to protect me. It is what she does best.

10

Hospitality Sweet

THE STORY IS TOLD of the cities of Sodom and
Gomorrah, notorious dens of iniquity, rife with
fornicators and homosexuals. God ordered the
destruction of these two cities and Abraham advocated
against collateral damage on their behalf. Less well
known about this oft-told tale is that it was not the sins of
promiscuity and buggery that angered God, but the sin
of being inhospitable. The ultimate mistreatment of
guests made God believe that these populations were
beyond redemption. Hospitality is a pillar of the Judeo-
Christian moral code of conduct. Every year at Passover
seder we repeat the Aramaic words "Kol Dichfin Yetay

v'yiphsach, Kol Ditsrich Yetay v'yochal"—"Let all who are weary come and rest. Let all who are hungry come and eat." It is a mitzvah, a good deed—the sort of thing for which karmic brownie points are awarded—but more than that, it is our civilized, human obligation. That's what I was taught growing up.

Ask anyone of my generation about the summer of 1967 and they are almost sure to speak of "the summer of love"—anyone except my family. For the Rakoffs it was clearly "the summer of hospitality." Free love? At our house it was free room-and-board. We were living in Montreal at the time and with Expo '67 in town, everybody my parents knew from around the globe—and some people they didn't really know—came to stay with us. My mother says that from May to August of that year we hosted 370 guest-nights. That's people in beds. That doesn't include meals served or the fact that one of the guests was my used-to-being-waited-upon grandmother, who stayed for six months.

My parents did not have a large house or very much money. What they did have were three children—six, four and two years old—jobs and busy lives. I don't believe it would have occurred to them to tell anybody they were not welcome to stay, that they were tired or overwhelmed. Nor would there have been any hesitation about feeding or entertaining all who graced our doorstep. Through my life I remember my mother saying, "A round table is better than a rectangle because you can always squeeze another chair around a circle." So, all who were weary came to rest and all who were hungry came to eat *chez* Rakoff.

For my brothers and me it felt like a constant party. We loved the comings and goings, the new faces, the relatives and friends from far-off lands. We even loved sharing our rooms and our beds. Bedtime became a nightly adventure necessitating complex negotiations about who would sleep where and with whom. Given that Simon, Davey and I were three of the smallest children ever invented, fitting two or sometimes three of us in a twin bed was easy. But it was when we got to share our beds with visiting children, experimenting to discover the most comfortable configurations, that nighttime became a real thrill. There was the two-pillows-two-heads-at-the-top-of-the-bed scenario, ideal for giggling. There was the mattress-separated-from-box-spring-and-put-on-the-floor scenario—perfect for acrobatics and trampolining. But my personal favorite was toes-meeting-toes-mid-mattress-with-a-head-at-either-end-of-the-bed; Doctor Dolittle's push-me pull-you, a two-headed llama of somebody's imagining that I believed actually existed until I was quite a lot older.

The magic of Expo '67 ended that summer, but my parents' hospitality to one and all did not. There was

Lauren, the troubled teenage daughter of dear friends who came to stay for a couple of weeks during a particularly difficult time in her life and ended up living with us on and off for years. There was Maurice, the young English lawyer who lived with us in Montreal, moved with us to Toronto and eventually got married in our house to Kathy, a woman to whom my mother introduced him. (It seemed my mother was running a full-service facility.) There was Ulrich, a Danish ballet dancer tenuously connected through friends of friends. Ulrich came for a few days while his U.S. visa was being sorted—and stayed several months, the velvet on one of his two pairs of tight trousers wearing thin and his honed muscles going soft. (The wooden banister of our staircase proved a poor substitute for a practice bar as the days accumulated.) Whole families of relatives arrived from South Africa and stayed until they found jobs and homes and lives. Students from abroad who lodged with us for academic terms, young doctors who boarded through medical rotations, and visiting professors whose quirks and idiosyncrasies were all accommodated.

Eventually, my parents had a bigger house and more money, but it was never about that. Add more water to the soup, stretch the stew with potatoes, turn a couch into a bed, stuff a pillowcase with an old sweatshirt. It was an attitude, a willingness. Two weddings, three bar mitzvahs (four if you count the one for my father on his forty-third birthday—a party thrown by my mother to quell Dad's stale refrains of having had a lesser bar mitzvah than his older brother, Julius—complete with a cake that read "Happy Bar Mitzvah Dad!"), a circumcision, endless parties and book club gatherings and dinners were all hosted in the home where I grew up. And so we learned to open our doors, our pantries and, yes, our beds to guests. We became externally social beings, platonic party sluts. My brothers and I can all cook, set a nice table, plate food esthetically and organize a shindig. There is always room for at least one more at my own round table, and as with my parents before me, I am not always sure how many teenagers may crawl out of my basement on any given morning. Breakfast is always served.

The concept of a bedroom as a private refuge is both relatively modern and predominantly Western. In other parts of the world, where space is at a premium, entertaining guests in one's bedchamber is the norm. When Tommy or I complain of our lack of space, which we sometimes do, we are quick to remind each other of some of the homes we have visited in less prosperous parts. Invited for a festive celebration at the home of Tommy's sitar teacher in Varanasi, we showed up on time, as is the custom in Canada, but not, as we discovered, in India. When we arrived, our host, not quite finished his afternoon nap, sat up in the bed that occupied a corner of the small house. Drowsy and disheveled, he muttered, "My problem, my one room." As couples and families are inclined to develop their own codes and dialects, this has entered our private lexicon. Griping about lack of space often elicits the response "My problem, my one room." We know how privileged we are.

In 1986, when Tommy and I moved to Tel Aviv, our friend Steve was spending the year in Jerusalem. Tel Aviv has a happening night life and club scene, whereas Jerusalem remains a spiritual pilgrimage center for Jews, Christians and Muslims alike. Though worlds apart in many significant ways, Tel Aviv and Jerusalem are only about a forty-five-minute bus ride from each other. We visited back and forth frequently during that year, more often than not spending the night. In truth, other than Friday nights, when buses don't run, we easily could have returned home on most occasions—Steve to Jerusalem or Tommy and I to Tel Aviv—but it was more fun to stay over. When the weather was fine, we preferred to congregate at our place in Tel Aviv for easy access to the beach, the bars and the clubs. But when the sun didn't shine, the Asiatic exoticism of Jerusalem was intoxicating.

Steve was renting a room in a flat in Rehavia, an upscale neighborhood within easy walking distance of downtown and the Old City. We spent many nights that winter strolling and exploring Jerusalem's nooks and crannies, and venturing into Arab neighborhoods that are no longer easily accessible or safe to wander late at night. Returning to Steve's flat after roaming the city, tired and chilled to the bone, we would settle down for the night.

The room he rented had at one time been the living room. It had been outfitted by the owner of the flat, probably around the time of the declaration of Israel's independence, with utilitarian *sochnut* furniture. In the early years of the State, the Sochnut (The Jewish Agency) would help facilitate new immigrants' absorption into their new homeland by providing a variety of services. Hebrew language instruction, employment services, interim housing and basic furniture were some of the perks of immigration to this hotbed of political strife for newcomers arriving from around the globe, often with nothing but the clothes on their backs.

Sochnut furniture was designed (and I use the term loosely) as a prime example of function over form— though if nothing else, it withstood the test of time. The room had a heavy wooden table that doubled as a desk and dining surface, a few mismatched wooden chairs, a bamboo and wicker bookshelf, an armoire with a blotchy mirror and a standard-issue *sochnut* bed-cum-chesterfield, proportionally ungenerous no matter what the function. Along the length of the bed, such as it was, was a thinly padded backrest upholstered in a dirty peach-colored faux brocade fabric. Matching the upholstery were two mattress cushions, one hard and thin, the other thicker but equally hard, that sat upon the plywood surface of the couch. The bed was no doubt designed according to Jewish law, which, as I have mentioned, values the mitzvah of welcoming guests into your home right up there with the Ten Commandments. Straddled beneath the metal bed frame was a second metal frame covered by a second plywood board. By pulling the bottom frame out from under the top frame and putting the thicker of the two mattresses on it, voilà, you had two beds—or, side by side, a somewhat meager double bed.

The three of us, Tommy, Steve and I, were not unfamiliar with sharing a bed. We had all met many years before at summer camp and through time had often slept in close quarters in large piles of sleeping-bagged adolescents in cabins, tents and parents' basements. It was a familiar and comfortable scenario. What was not comfortable was Steve's bed. Only marginally wider than a couple of army cots and barely more cushioned, it required cooperation from all co-slumbering participants. In order for the three of us to fit on the platform, we all needed to lie on our sides facing the same direction. The

WHEN MY WORLD WAS VERY SMALL

middle was the prized position because although one lay on the crevice, one was also less likely to be pushed out of bed during the night—though even that provided no guarantee. If anyone wanted to roll over and face the other direction he or she would shout in their best impersonation of an old Eastern European Jew "Svitch!" and we would comply and switch positions in unison. It was far from an ideal situation, but it was a choice. We were young enough to not care too much about a solid night's sleep.

After one such night in Jerusalem, Steve woke up feeling a little melancholy. I believe he was suffering from sleep deprivation more than anything.

"I wish I had a real bed," he declared. "A real queen-size bed."

"It's probably not so bad when we're not here," I said, trying to cheer him up.

"Ya, but then it's just a crappy, skimpy bed. A queen-size bed is more than just a bed. It's an event."

I knew exactly what he meant.

At least I thought I knew.

It wasn't until years later, when I got sick, that I truly understood the concept of a bed as a venue, a social happening, an occasion for hospitality.

While some people might be inclined to retreat into solitude in times of crisis, my instinct was for company.

Granted, it was grossly self-indulgent to presume that anyone would want to hang out with me during my illness, given my less-than-scintillating conversational ability, my depressing circumstance and the pathetic visual specimen that I was. That said, all the tweaking my fabulous friends had done to make my bedroom a comfortable place in which to convalesce had inadvertently made it an inviting place to hang out.

Coming to visit while I recovered from surgery, my friend Ian climbed the stairs to my bedroom and sat down in the chair next to my bed. We chatted briefly while I lay there, and then out of the blue, belying his polite Anglo upbringing, Ian said, "You do look so comfortable. I think I'll join you." And swift as a kitten, he did. And I was delighted to have him.

As it happened that day, our conversation turned to sex. I don't recall exactly how or why, but we got on the topic of teaching teens about safe sex and the importance thereof and I said, "I believe it's an unrealistic and impossible task. They don't believe they are mortal, so how can you get the message through that there is something out there that can harm them?"

"What do you mean 'they don't believe they're mortal'?" Ian, having had no cause to face his own mortality, didn't understand.

"None of us do. Not really. Death is something that

happens eventually. We know that rationally, but emotionally, we don't really see it in our own futures. Serious illness happens to other people—not to us. Until you face it head-on, I mean like when it actually happens to you, you don't really believe it can or will. And that's how most adults feel. We are all immortal despite the inevitability of death. For teens, that sense of eventually is so far removed, they think they are invincible. Safe sex, hell, safe *anything* doesn't seem to apply to them."

"I'm not sure I agree," Ian said. Somehow his discongruity fed my delusion that if my guests felt comfortable enough to get in my bed and at the same time disagree with me, I was not completely failing as a hostess. I was thoroughly relieved that he didn't feel he had to agree with me just because I had cancer. If only I could muster the energy to whip up some refreshments . . .

Ian wasn't the only one to climb into my bed. I have no intention of outing everyone who cuddled under my covers (you know who you are), but there did seem to be some sort of organic force at work. Maybe it was the brightly colored bed linens or the fluffy pillows. Perhaps people were unconsciously seduced by sweet-smelling remnants left in my bed from my children's snacks or maybe my medication-soaked body emitted narcotic enticements that encouraged snuggling. Having never in my life felt less sexy, paradoxically it had never been easier to get people into bed with me.

When Steve and Tracey and their son Oscar said they were coming from Calgary over Christmas holidays, I knew their visit would be a wonderful elixir to counteract the debilitating effects of chemotherapy. When our Steve first met Tracey, one of the reasons we loved her right away was that she was happy to go along with all or at least most of the silly games we'd been playing together for years. Because we live far apart, our usual pattern when we are lucky enough to have time together is to eat too much, laugh too hard, drink to excess, stay up too late and generally regress to adolescence. We can sleep when the party is over!

By the time the holidays rolled around I had finished four of my eight rounds of "dense dose" chemotherapy. I had no hair and had so far lost close to twenty pounds. I wasn't in bed all the time—sometimes I was on the couch. On good days I could eat and even go out for a bit, but my energy was very limited. Nonetheless, there was a party to be had and I had no intention of missing it. More importantly, there would be guests in my home and it was my responsibility to host them respectably. Could I show my guests a good time? I knew that was not why they were coming for a visit, but I was also aware that this was their holiday.

"Bring pajamas," I told them over the phone. "We have housecoats and slippers."

Though I didn't do the shopping myself, I made sure the house was stocked with appropriately decadent and fun treats and snacks. Tracey has a sweet tooth, so there were chocolates and cookies and ice cream. Tommy is a salty snacker, so chips and other crunchies were available. And Steve, when he's around us, likes "treif," forbidden fruit, specifically pork and pork products. Wine and beer and scotch and soft drinks, tea and coffee and a wide variety of take-out menus were all on hand. Pillows and blankets and soft cozy throws and movies and whole seasons of television shows were all stockpiled so we could hunker down together.

Each night, by the time we were through dinner, I was worn out. "I'm going up to bed. Come keep me company," I would say. And when the dishes had been done and the leftovers put away and the children were engaged in some activity or another, one by one the adults would arrive and make themselves comfortable in my chamber. Trays and glasses and bottles and bowls of treats in hand, Tracey and Steve and Tommy would climb the stairs ready to bring the party to me rather than demanding that I join them.

And when I had consumed my festive tea and could not sustain any more conversation nor keep my body vertical nor my eyes open, they would notice that I was fading and say, "You're tired. We'll go downstairs now."

"No, stay," I would say. "I don't want to miss anything."

With my queen-size bed full of people who I love quietly conversing or watching a movie, I would drift off to sleep, assured that while I was not the life of the party, I was still a gracious host, my bed an event.

11

I'm Number One!

FOR A BRIEF PERIOD right at the beginning my mind was stuck at "I am willing to do what it takes to get rid of this." I knew that it would be brutal, but I don't think it really occurred to me that one of the possibilities still was death. I think after I got my "good news, stage II cancer" report I somehow thought I was in the clear. I forgot I was still at risk. The doctors reminded me regularly.

When I had met with my oncologist the day before starting chemotherapy I had been like a swollen river overflowing with questions about my future. They were important, well-thought-out questions. For instance, if

I chose down the road to have a prophylactic mastectomy on the other side, would I be eliminating a potential early warning signal? My thinking was as follows: Breast cancer is a primary cancer. As long as it's in the breast tissue or lymph nodes, it is treatable, with statistically good outcomes if found early enough. Metastatic breast cancer spreads to the bones or liver. Once that happens, it is incurable. This is what I surmised from previous oncological encounters and sporadic reading. Therefore, finding breast cancer at the primary stage, meaning in the breast as opposed to in the bones or liver, is actually a good thing on the cancer scale. Ergo, if you remove a healthy breast to prevent cancer, which may or may not occur at some later date, is it like sending the miners down the shaft without the canary?

"Stop thinking," my oncologist had said to me. "While your question, despite its lack of medically sound information, is certainly an interesting one, the process that led you to it is no doubt exhausting. Conserve your resources to face the impending challenges of chemotherapy."

And yet, the sickness, the weakness and the brain-numbing effects of the treatments could not shut down my own personal panic-processing plant.

"Should I have a prophylactic mastectomy on the other side?" I asked my breast surgeon.

"I can't make that decision for you," she replied.

"I don't want you to make that decision for me. I just want your input. Based on your knowledge and experience, what would you do?"

"My experience is all secondhand. I haven't had breast cancer. It's a very personal decision." The professional, cover-your-ass response.

"Should I have a prophylactic mastectomy on the other side?" I asked my oncologist again at an appointment about halfway through my eight rounds of chemotherapy.

"Well, statistically, it wouldn't affect your outcomes either way."

"Statistically." Except I didn't want stats. I wanted input. I wanted human, emotional, "what would you do if it was you, your mother, your wife, your daughter" opinions.

I tried to speak his language.

"Statistically, I've heard that one in nine women will get breast cancer, correct?"

"That's what the fund-raisers say," he replied.

"What does that mean?" I asked, suppressing a what-the-*fuck*-does-that-mean tone.

"Well, before age ninety, one in nine women will get breast cancer. In other words, if they live long enough, statistically, one in nine women will get breast cancer."

"Okay," I said, "on my right side, I'm one—as in, I'm already statistically the one of the nine. So what does that make my left breast, statistically?"

"What do you mean?" he asked, becoming confused by my neurosis-induced reasoning.

"Let's talk probability. Before my diagnosis, I had a one-in-nine probability of getting cancer before I turned ninety. Now, knowing what we know, I have gone from a probability of approximately 11 percent, to a probability of 100 percent. I am 100 percent sure to have breast cancer in my right breast. So, given that I'm nowhere near ninety years old, and as you yourself have told me I'm 'statistically' about twenty years too young for my diagnosis, where does that leave my left breast? I fell victim to the odds once, so am I now one in five, or one in six, or am I still one in nine?"

"I can tell you that the cancer you already had will not spread to your other breast. That's not how it works. At least not the kind of breast cancer you had. What I cannot tell you is where it came from in the first place. I don't know if you are more prone to breast cancer than the statistically average person other than to say that since you have already had it you are obviously susceptible in some way."

The prophylactic mastectomy question got lost in the shuffle of statistics and supposition—again.

"What would be the reasons to go ahead with a prophylactic mastectomy?" I asked my breast surgeon at my next visit.

"It wouldn't prevent a recurrence of this cancer," she non-answered.

"I know. So why would one do it?" I switched to the theoretical "one" thinking that a hypothetical patient might get a more direct response.

"Cosmetically, the results of reconstruction tend to be more satisfying when both breasts are done. It is very difficult to match a reconstructed breast to a natural breast. If you get the breast surgeon and the plastic surgeon to operate during the same procedure, it's only one anesthetic. Also, some patients find it provides peace of mind. It's not a guarantee, but it eliminates some of the anxiety for some people."

At last. The surgeon had used my magic words. "Eliminates anxiety." I sighed. It was suddenly clear to me what to ask.

"Why would one choose not to go ahead with a prophylactic mastectomy if one were opting for reconstruction anyhow?" I saw the light go on in her eyes. Somehow I had phrased the question in such a way that she could answer it safely.

"As you already know, recovery from a mastectomy requires drains, and rehabilitation of the affected arm. Some people would rather avoid that. Some women prefer to keep their remaining breast to maintain natural sensation, in some cases contributing to greater sexual

satisfaction. I guess those would be the cons to prophylactic mastectomy."

"Thank you." That was good enough for me. Reduction
of anxiety versus nipple stimulation felt like a no-
brainer. "When can we book the surgery?"

The breast surgeon and I agreed that having a pre-operative
mammogram would be useful to avoid any surprises during
surgery or from the post-operative pathology report. I was
understandably agitated. My previous "routine" mammogram had unveiled the shocking presence of the cancer
lurking within me. What if my body was about to ambush
me again? What if the chemo hadn't killed all the cancer
cells? What if . . . ? What if . . . ? What if . . . ?

I what-iffed myself into a panicked frenzy. I decided
to go to my mammogram appointment alone, subscrib-
ing to the old dictum of facing one's fears head-on.
I recalled, however, that this notion had something to
do with the treatment of phobias—irrational fears—
which was hardly what I was facing. I had every reason
in the world to be frightened. An annual mammogram
was what you underwent to be sure there was no cancer,
not what you did to discover that there was.

The waiting room at the breast screening center
was full. A variety of women wearing street clothes from
the waist down, topped by pale blue hospital gowns, sat

in a state of naive suspension leafing through ancient magazines. I noted no hats, no wigs, nor any short hair. They all appeared to be older than me and there for routine screening.

The elderly woman volunteering on that day glanced at my chart and handed me a gown.

"You know the drill," she said lightheartedly.

I smiled and nodded, as though my familiarity with the process was like membership in a secret society. I took the gown and made my way to one of the curtained cubicles.

As I drew the curtain closed, the feeling hit me like a tidal wave—unanticipated, unprocessed turmoil engulfed me. My knees buckled, and the small bench at the edge of the cubicle caught me on the way down. I couldn't strip from the waist up and go into that waiting room full of women. Removing my bra meant removing my prosthetic breast. Beneath the loose cloth of the hospital gown my obvious amputation would be on display. Nobody waiting for a mammogram wants to be confronted by the worst-case scenario.

The waiting room volunteer lady may have wondered why I took so long to emerge from the change room, but if so, she gave no indication of this. I went and sat in the waiting room, self-conscious that everybody was surely aware that I still had my bra on, a clear trespass of the mammogram code of conduct. Ironic that, I of all people was suddenly concerned with breaking rules, not to mention convinced that everybody was undoubtedly paying close attention to my brassiere and me. Hanging on the wall opposite where I sat was a poster of two mammogram images side by side—one quite clear and sharp, the other blurry and difficult to see. Underneath the photographs was a caption that said something like, "This is why we squeeze so hard" and a brief explanation that the tighter the mammography plates hugged the flesh of the breast, the better the resulting image. Each year I had read this poster before going in to have my breasts sandwiched, squeezed and x-rayed, and each year it had made sense to me. Now more than ever I wanted to feel the pain so there would be no doubt or uncertainty.

The mammographer didn't say anything when I took an extra moment to remove my bra and silicon stuffing prior to having my one remaining breast—not long for this world—sandwiched between the sheets of Plexiglas. As the machine squeezed my flesh, it was not dread or fear that I felt, but unwavering conviction that proceeding with the second mastectomy was the right decision for me. I'd do anything to avoid being number one ever again.

12

Toads, Snails, Puppy Dog
Tails and Pizza

S AFI WAS THE FIRST. The others were all out of
the house and he came to snuggle with me in bed,
a weekend morning ritual that both of us are
still reluctant to give up. As we lay there on that late
winter day, Safi asked, "What did they take off you?
Your kidney?"

My surgery had coincided with a friend's kidney
donation, so his confusion was understandable. I had
spent many mental moments preparing for this occasion
and replied without hesitation, "No, it was my breast that
was removed."

"Really?" Safi said, sounding shocked and dismayed.

"Yes," I said, "but that's why I will be having another operation, so they can build me a new one."

"How do you build a breast?" he asked.

"Well, it'll be kind of like a water balloon in my chest," I tried to explain.

"Do you get to choose the color?" he asked.

"What color?"

"Of the balloon," he said.

"No, it's not an actual balloon. It's like a balloon, but it will be under my skin. You won't be able to see it or tell it isn't real," I answered, trying not to laugh. But I couldn't help remembering a time when the boys had shoved balloons under their T-shirts and marched around the house chanting, *"We have ladies' boobies, we have ladies' boobies."* No wonder Safi was confused.

He thought about it for a moment and started to get out of my bed.

"Are you leaving because what I told you frightened you? Does it make you uncomfortable?" I asked.

"No," he replied.

"I'd like you to stay for a while," I said, trying hard not to sound needy or desperate.

"Okay," he said, reentering our shared cocoon of pillows and blankets and warmth.

I hugged him, and kissed him, and tickled him, just like a mother with two breasts.

—

It wasn't long before my cancer diplomacy skills were once again put to the test. Amit was the second of the children to broach the subject of my missing breast. Safi and Amit share a bedroom, and much to Safi's chagrin Amit sings himself to sleep every night. Standing next door in Micah's bedroom, as I sorted neatly folded laundry into the chaotic cupboard, I could hear Amit beginning his nightly solo at full volume.

"I'm a Barbie Girl
In a Barbie World
It's fantastic
My boobs are plastic!"

"That's not funny!" Safi said indignantly.

"It is funny." Amit refrained, *"It's fantastic / My boobs are plastic!"*

"I don't think it's funny," Safi said with seriousness belying his youth. "Mom has plastic breasts."

"No, she doesn't."

"Yes, she does."

"No, she doesn't."

"Yes, she does."

"Mawwwwm!"

"Yes," I said, appearing quickly in their bedroom.

"Safi says you have plastic breasts. Is that true?" Amit asked with the confidence of an older brother assured of his superiority of knowledge and experience.

"Well, actually, I have one real breast," I said, self-consciously nonchalant.

"How can you have only one breast?" he asked, genuinely curious.

"Well"—I cleared my throat—"when I had the operation to remove the cancer, there was so much of it that to make sure they got it all out and give me the best chance of never having to go through any of this again, they had to remove my whole breast." Did he believe the calm I willed myself to project? Could he hear my heart pounding through my silicone prosthesis?

"Oh. So how come you still look like you have two breasts?" Amit asked, ever the logical thinker.

"Well, I have a fake one I wear in my bra." I paused, leaving space for more questions.

"Oh," he said.

There was a long silence. I started to move toward the door.

"Can you lie in my bed?" Amit asked, stifling a yawn.

"Sure," I said, relieved.

I climbed onto the mountain of layers he had created for himself from blankets, plush toys and clothes destined for the hamper. Rocking my hips from side to side I wedged a place for myself in the crook of his body. Laying my head close to his, I could hear his breath, nasal and noisy, begin to slow. The warmth from his cheeks demanded an unsolicited kiss. I watched his eyelids flicker in the darkness, giving way to the acceptance of sleep. Rolling toward the edge of the bed I gently placed my feet on the floor and silently made my exit.

Two down, one to go. With Safi and Amit in the know, I was sure it wouldn't be long before Micah would hear the news about my fake breast through the grapevine.

It didn't happen.

It was as though the brothers had, for the first time ever, taken a vow of secrecy. Just when I thought their naturally loose lips would save me from having to bring up the subject of my breasts *again* with my teenage son, Amit and Safi were mute.

It had nothing to do with embarrassment. With me leading the pack, our household had become breast-obsessed since my diagnosis. Following my mastectomy, as a means of coping with my grief, I began compulsively sculpting tiny breasts from an oven-bake modeling material. Dozens and dozens of miniature replicas of my right breast and axila were painstakingly formed, with contrasting color of nipple and areola, baked, lacquered, and mounted on brooch pins. I gave them away to friends who visited, neighbors who brought meals—anybody I thought might humor me and pin my breast to their clothing.

I reasoned that if I wasn't sporting my right breast, everybody else I knew could wear it for me.

"How many breasts are you making, Mom?"

"As many as I have to," I replied.

"I saw Claudia wearing your breast, Mom."

"Simon says he wants one of your breasts, Mom."

The subject was far from *taboob*. And yet, despite the constant talk about my breasts, and Safi's and Amit's knowledge of my "single" status, Micah remained in the dark and uniquely uninterested. Holding my breath in anticipation of his eventual query was exhausting. I would have to tell him, if only to clear a path for me to process other real, and imaginary, problems and pitfalls. This one was obscuring my view of the horizon.

Over the Easter break, we went to a small family reunion in Niagara Falls. Two grandparents, two aunts, two uncles and six cousins all together at the Hilton Niagara Falls for a fun-filled weekend. It was my idea. I was still recovering from aggressive chemo, and this seemed like a better way to spend time with the clan than having them all come to stay with us in Toronto. We booked a hotel with a pool and a three-story waterslide on the assumption that while I napped, everyone else could play. I wanted to participate but just didn't have the energy to go full steam. So, off they went to explore the pool, while I recharged my batteries in our room.

When I awoke, the troops had not returned. I went to look for them at the pool. They were ecstatically engaged in boisterous games and competitions of breath-holding stamina, somersaults, handstands and sliding down the three-story, corkscrew waterslide. Cheering each other on as they reached the final precipice and careened off the edge, splashing into the chlorine bath, they were as happy as could be.

I stood by the edge of the pool observing a level of energy and enthusiasm I couldn't muster. When my family eventually noticed me, they shrilled for my attention and participation.

"Mom! Mom! Watch this!"

"Mom! Are you coming in?"

"Mom! Watch me come down the slide!"

"Mom! Go put on your bathing suit!"

"Mom! You gotta try the slide!"

"Ya, Mom! Come on the slide!"

"Let's get Mom on the slide!"

Micah began the chant. "Slide! Slide! Slide . . . !"

The others joined in. "Slide! Slide! Slide!"

I slunk away, embarrassed by their good-natured prodding, and returned to my room. With no hair and one breast, I was not going to frolic in a public swimming pool. I could barely stand to look at myself in the privacy of my own bathroom. But I feared my children—especially Micah—would see me as a stick-in-the-mud. Once again the cogs of my brain took on an adrenaline-induced fervor as I determined just the right approach to take.

When the kids returned from the pool I took Micah aside.

"When you're dried and dressed, I'd like to talk to you," I said, attempting a casual tone.

"Okay. Is it serious?"

"Well, I need to talk to you about one serious thing, and one not-serious thing, but it can wait till you're dressed."

Safi and Amit were happily occupied in my brother-in-law's hotel room, channel surfing with their cousins—a novel and exciting activity for children deprived of cable TV. I waited for Micah to emerge from the bathroom.

"So what did you want to tell me, Mom?" Micah asked, perching on the edge of the bed as he fiddled with the television remote.

"Well, as I said, I have one serious, and one not-serious thing I need to talk to you about. Please turn off the TV and give me three minutes of undivided attention." I gently removed the remote control from Micah's hand.

"When I had the operation to remove the cancer from my breast, there was so much disease in the tissue that it was necessary to remove the entire breast. Did you know that already?"

"No, I didn't. I hadn't really thought about it."

Typical teenager. If it wasn't about him, it wasn't on his radar.

"Well, in place of a real breast, I have a fake one that fits in a pocket in my bra. I have a bathing suit with a pocket, but even if I felt like swimming, which I don't, there is no way I would get on that twisty slide. I'd come swirling down the slide, splashing into the pool, and my boob would fly out into the water like a lopsided beach-ball." I giggled nervously. "So, it's just not happening. I will not be joining you in the water this weekend. Okay?"

"Okay. So what's the serious thing?" Micah asked.

"That's it," I said, relieved that it had gone so easily. "The not-serious thing is that the adults would like you, as the oldest of the cousins, to babysit the others tonight. We want to order pizza for all the kids, get a pay-per-view movie, and have you be in charge while we go to dinner at the restaurant in the hotel."

"You mean *we're* having pizza and *you're* going to a fancy restaurant?" He promptly burst into sobs.

"I just told you that I had my entire breast lopped off because of cancer and you're crying about pizza?" I exclaimed with utter disbelief.

As I handed back the television remote to my son, it occurred to me that food was something he could relate to. Breasts, not so much.

13

Cancer Club

LLOWING THE SIDE DOOR of the garage to open no more than a crack, the pudding-y boy peeked out at me from the darkness through his grease-smudged, thick glasses.

"What's the password?" he asked in the most menacing tone he could muster.

Compared to my slight, six-year-old frame he appeared monolithic. His box-like mass, wedged into the ungenerous opening, blocked my view of the inner sanctum of the garage where the big kids were hanging out.

"What password?" I asked.

"The clubhouse password," he barked.

"I dunno? Can I come in?" I asked innocently, knowing just enough to try to disguise my welling sense of intimidation. "I need to talk to my brother."

"Who's your brother?"

"Simon," I replied, more meekly than I had intended.

Closing the door almost all the way, so that only the tips of his fingers gripping the edge of the doorjamb were still visible, I heard the boy speak like the naughty boys who became donkeys in Pinocchio. "Hey, Simon! It's your kid sista. She says she has ta talk to you."

The big kids—all the eight- and nine-year-olds from the block—had been holed up in a neighbor's garage for hours. I didn't particularly care what they were doing, I just knew I desperately wanted to be included.

"Does she know the password?" I heard my brother's voice from the depths of the cinder-block cavern.

Before the door was edged open again, I could feel my throat tightening. The shock of my brother's public betrayal of our filial bond stung like a giant belly flop. Simon, two years my elder, was not malicious. Small for his age, clumsy, uncoordinated and blind in one eye, he was used to being either picked on or ignored by kids his own age. We played together always—him finding it easier to keep up physically with a younger sister than with his peers—me never mocking him when he failed to keep up. But here he was, my ally, my pal, turning against me.

"He wants to know if you know the password?" echoed the plump boy, peering down at me through the meager opening.

I tried to stop the tears from escaping, but as I opened my mouth to speak it was as though a cork had been removed and the fluid began spilling from my eyes and nose. Wiping the inflating bubbles of snot with the back of my hand, leaving snail trails smeared halfway up my skinny arm, I sputtered, "I jjjjust nnneed to talk ttttto mmmm Simon."

The nine-year-old border guard, surprised and defeated by my blubbering, opened the door halfway. Looking backwards over his shoulder toward the other kids he asked, "Hey, guys, should we tell her the password?"

A group of six or seven bored-looking boys and girls sat on the cement floor amid piles of smooth, shiny, dark brown chestnuts and discarded, thorny chestnut casings. Sensing a diversion from the tedium of sorting and trading chestnuts—the autumn preoccupation of the neighborhood children—the big kids moved toward the open door. Simon, unsure of the popular sentiment in play, was last to appear at the entrance.

"Ya, let's tell her," said one of the kids.

I was pleased that my crying had had an unanticipated positive effect. I managed to quell my tears and reduce the stream of snot to a sniffle. In unison, the children chanted slowly, "One . . . two . . . three." And then, all together they rattled off the password so loud and so fast that it sounded like a clattering freight train. When they had finished, they burst into collective peals of laughter, knowing full well that I couldn't possibly have gleaned enough information to grant my entry into the club.

"Slower," I shouted at my tormentors.

"Okay," said one of the bigger girls. "Chinesechika-daioongapoongawillywillywaxa."

I turned and walked away seething with frustration, anger and the stabbing pain of treason.

When Simon came home, he tried, out of earshot of my mother, to taunt me with rapid-fire repetitions of the club password.

"Chinesechikadaioongapoongawillywillywaxachi-nesechikadaioongapoongawillywillywaxachinesechi-kadaioongapoongawillywillywaxa."

But by then, I didn't care.

"Who cares about your stupid club anyhow," I said. And I meant it.

I couldn't articulate why I didn't care, but something had altered my desire to belong. The full-body response to being so obviously not wanted had shifted my tides.

Simon was incensed. His deep black eyes opened wide with disbelief beneath his tuft of unruly black hair. His shoulders curled forward, his hips dropped and his soft, round belly protruded as though some powerful post that had been propping him upright had begun to melt.

Pushing one knock-knee forward in an attempt to assume a more powerful stance, he whined, "Hey, Ruthie, I'm in the club and you're not," in a nya-nya singsong.

Nothing good ever came of that tone.

"So," I replied.

"Don't you want to be in the club?"

"Nope," I said.

Completely bamboozled by this rapid loss of lordship over his little sister, Simon begged, "Please let me teach you the password."

"Nah," I replied.

"Come on, pal," he repeated, patting me on the head with a gently bouncing, stiff hand—a different secret password understood only by our sibling triumvirate.

So, to restore our usual camaraderie to its natural order, I let him.

Slowly, precisely, Simon chanted, "Chinese chickadai, oonga poonga, willy willy waxa."

I have never forgotten the password.

Shortly after the password incident, I was denied entry into another club. It was late in the afternoon, and I was playing at my friend Irish's house.

"It's time for Ruth to go home now," her mother called upstairs.

"Aw, does she have to? Can't she stay for dinner?" Irish shouted down to her mother.

"Not tonight, dear," Irish's mother replied in a tighter tone.

Making her way to the top of the staircase, Irish asked, "Why not?"

"Because," her mother responded.

"Because why?" Irish asked, not picking up on her mother's mounting irritation.

"Because we are going to the club," said her mother with finality.

There it was again, that word. *Club.* I had no idea at what club one might have dinner, and I was intrigued.

"Can't Ruth come with us to the club?" Irish asked, bounding down the stairs in little leaps, using the banister as a crutch-cum-pole vault.

"No, she cannot," I heard her mother say.

Irish, still unwilling to take no for an answer, responded with another "Why not?"

"Because she's Jewish," was what I heard from my perch at the top of the stairs.

I wasn't shocked or offended. I really had no inkling as to what going to a club and being Jewish had to do with each other. All I knew was that I no longer had even the slightest interest in going to that club, or any club.

So, at the tender age of six, with next to no knowledge of clubs other than as entities with a propensity to exclude me, I became a non-joiner. I would never belong to a glee club, a drama club, or a chess club. I would never sign up for a country club, a yacht club, or a health club. It didn't concern me who would have me or who wouldn't. And that was that.

—

Those many years later, when I was nervously waiting for the biopsy results of the lump that had been found in my right breast, I was thoroughly exhausted by the doing-nothing of it. I can scarcely think of anything more passive than waiting. Waiting for the light to change—not walking or driving, but waiting. Waiting for the movie to start—not getting ready to go, not getting there, not buying tickets, or lining up for popcorn—waiting. It is anti-doing.

What I did not realize at the time was that I was, in fact, doing something quite profound. I was inadvertently going through a rigorous initiation into a not-nearly-exclusive-enough club. I was on the path to the cancer club. The steps include, but are not limited to, the classic Kübler-Ross grief roller coaster of shock, denial, anger, bargaining, depression, testing and acceptance. Add to these the lesser-known rights of passage of distraction, narcissism, tribalism and re-normalization—and presto, you're a member.

Had it not been for the unyielding attentions of my friends, the doing-nothing of waiting might have paralyzed me completely. Ironically, doing something is far easier than doing nothing.

I assume there was a great deal of planning and coordinating going on behind my back. There must have been. But, I had lost my wide-angle lens on life and could perceive only a narrow corridor of activity that involved me directly, having unwittingly entered a realm of narcissism the likes of which I could not previously have fathomed. Was Tommy calling my friends while he was at work, making sure they were checking up on me? Were my friends calling one another to coordinate who would occupy me when? All I knew was that there was a flurry of activity in my direction.

There were endless invitations for walks in the mornings and afternoons. There were stupid, mindless movies attended in large adolescent-like packs. There were manufactured important shopping excursions. There were lunches and matinees. There were late-night visits to my rooftop deck to chat and hang out. All of it shrouded by the pretense that we were simply doing what we always did.

But it was not what we had always done. Cathy did not usually zip me around town midday, midweek in her convertible, with the top down, feigning carefree with a fervor that can only be generated by tremendous effort. Iris did not usually have time in her busy workday for leisurely lunches and tours of the new theater complex she was managing. And Kate had never before taken me for a pedicure at the Vietnamese nail salon.

In fact, I had never been to one of these assembly line salons before under any circumstances. But there I was, an active participant in the "let's have fun" charade, playing the role of Lady of Leisure. Rows of pedicure chairs—each equipped with remote-controlled, electric massage capabilities and a foot bath—each attended by a small, attractive, young Vietnamese woman. Hundreds of bottles of colored nail lacquer lining the walls, each with a suitably irreverent name to describe its shade. "Friar, Friar, Pants on Fire." "Princesses Rule!" "Miso Happy with this Color."

Incapable of decision making in my current state, I removed the small bottles one by one from the shelf, turning each over to read the name out loud.

"'Sea? I Told You,' 'Keys to My Karma,' 'Call My Cellery,'" I read before carefully replacing each bottle.

"That would be a fun job," I said to Kate. "Being the person who got to make up the names for nail colors or paint shades."

The salon's boss, a wolf-like little man who paced back and forth between the parallel rows of treatment thrones, shot my pedicurist a piercing glance. She hurried over to where I was standing.

"This one very nice color," she said, snatching one of the small bottles from beneath my caressing fingers. "You choose this one."

Pleased that someone else had made yet another decision for me, I agreed. She raced me back to my chair and hustled me through my pedicure so that the chair could be filled with someone new as fast as possible.

While my friends occupied me and coddled me, some of them suggested that perhaps I should get in touch with support groups available to people dealing with cancer. I wasn't interested. Just because I had cancer didn't mean I had to join any cancer clubs. I was doing just fine with all the support I had *outside* the cancer community.

As I had drifted in and out of post-surgical consciousness after my mastectomy, Raziel, an old family friend, appeared with a bouquet of exquisite cream-colored roses. Raziel had at that time just recently finished treatments for bladder cancer. Other than immediate family, he was my only visitor in hospital. He knew I belonged before I was even aware that there was a club. The flowers he brought were not the usual get-well-soon offering, but a sad welcome gift, a token of shared experience. Welcome to the cancer clan!

As the parameters of my old world got smaller—no bigger in fact than the space I took up in bed or on the couch—my new world began to include everybody who had or *had* had their own cancer. It turns out that membership in the cancer club isn't optional.

I am not comfortable with the term *survivor*. To me a survivor is someone who went through the Holocaust. Also, I can't help thinking that the term *survivor*, worn as it is like a badge of honor, somehow implies something negative about those who do not survive, those who succumb— that they are somehow lesser, weaker, not entitled to a moniker of victory. Instead, I have been toying with some sort of "journey" or "traveler" metaphor, but as yet have not found exactly the right fit. It occurs to me that *survivor* implies the journey is over, and I'm not sure it ever completely is. An alcoholic is always an alcoholic even after decades of sobriety and thousands of AA meetings. At this stage I can't imagine my journey through cancer ever ceasing to color or inform who I am, who I have become. Perhaps I simply haven't arrived yet.

That said, membership in the cancer club gives one tunnel vision. Once you are in, a poignant awareness of other members emerges. It is not type specific. Despite the uniqueness of each diagnosis and every experience, the universal bond that determines club membership defies cell permutations and mutations. Slowly, my belonging became apparent to me.

Out for lunch with a friend, I noticed a woman wearing a close-fitting cap. It was a cold day, so to the uninitiated it may simply have appeared to be weather- or fashion-related, but not to me. I knew she was one of us. She looked at me, and I looked at her. We didn't smile or wink at each other in any discernible way. It was silent acknowledgment from one capped woman to another. I wondered if she noticed that we both ate only half our food. I wondered if she wondered about me what I wondered about her—what kind, what stage, what grade?

I bump into James, an acquaintance, in the street. My belonging to the club is unmistakable at the height of treatments.

"Are you doing cancer?" James asks.

"Yup, I'm doing cancer," I reply, knowing that he is a fellow traveler.

"What kind?" James asks.

"Breast," I say.

"Lung," he says, gripping my shoulder as though it is a secret handshake.

"Keep the faith," he says, and moves on.

People who are not members of the cancer club want to introduce members to each other. "This is Debbie. She also had breast cancer."

Or they assume that membership implies association. "You must know Ginny. She had breast cancer."

And to my surprise, I want to meet Debbie and I will seek out Ginny now that I know they are members. We are bound together by shared experience, by catastrophe, by hope.

People also feel compelled to share with me stories of friends or loved ones who belong to the club, presuming I will care. And they are right. I do care. More than I know. I want to hear the good-news stories of people five years out or ten years out. I also need to hear the bad-news stories so I do not lose sight of the horrifying possibilities that are my reality. So I remember why I am submitting to surgery and treatments that feel as though they will kill me.

My friend Dionie visits and tells me about her cousin, recently diagnosed.

"What kind of cancer?" I ask.

"Sinus cancer," Dionie replies.

"Is she having treatment?"

"No. I don't think there is any treatment," she says, tearing up.

"How old is she?" I need to know.

"Thirty-four."

"And there is nothing that can be done?" I want to protest, march, rally—I just don't know where.

"No. There is nothing that can be done."

"Is she married? Does she have kids? Is she working?" I want information. I need information. As though knowing about another member of the club can help either of us.

"She worked in a nail salon, but she can't anymore," Dionie says.

We both know that what is unsaid is that cancer is killing her cousin and we both feel the sadness of kin.

As a member of the club, cancer greets one in the most unexpected places. Another day I return to the Vietnamese nail salon for a manicure and pedicure. I have decided I am worthy of a treat. My nails are disintegrating from my chemotherapy treatments. I want to cover them with polish so I do not have to see the bruises and scars. As I enter, the toxic smell of the acetones and polishes accosts my olfactory nerves. Near the front of the salon, a woman with impossibly long fingernails talks too loudly on her cell phone. A small Vietnamese woman leans in close to the woman's unoccupied hand and airbrushes an intricate pattern onto each nail. The atmosphere is prickly and acrid and I can taste the chemicals on my tongue. These are the poisons that are killing Dionie's cousin, I theorize with revulsion.

The boss, overseeing his business, trying to eke out a living in a new country, might as well have horns and a pointy tail. I see him as a pimp, selling the services of the young women in his employ. He is not selling their bodies, their sex—only their sinuses are being sacrificed on his altar. I want to scream, "Run, get out while you can! Save yourselves! Go back to your villages! Return to your families!" But they are not members of the tribe. They would not understand. And me, I have lost the strength of character that would in the past have allowed, nay, *compelled* me to voice my opinion and behave with conscience. I sit down in the chair to which I am led and partake in the multicolored biohazard seduction.

Raziel and I speak on the phone and share tips about managing nausea and medication.

"Have you been eating?" we ask one another.

And sometimes we answer "yes" and sometimes "no."

"You should try a Gravol suppository about twenty minutes before taking domperidone. Then an Ondanse-tron chaser," I suggest to him. I have learned the lingo only too well.

Raziel recommends an outing to see the beautiful cherry blossoms in High Park. He knows it will be good for me to leave my couch (which has developed a divot distinctly reminiscent in size and shape to my hindquarters). Because he holds more seniority in the club, I heed his advice, defer to his guidance. We go at dusk, on a beautiful spring evening—the kind that banishes winter and beckons summer—my parents, my children and I. There we are along with what seem to be all the Japanese residents of the city standing beneath a vast canopy of white flowers. The late-day sunlight streams through the branches and bounces off the pond at the bottom of the hill, reflecting back on to the cherry blossoms, turning the white petals to iridescent pearls that cling to craggy branches. The children climb the trees. Endless, androgynous Japanese boys pose for photographs. One sublimely elegant woman, in honey-colored linen and beautiful, high, pointy cream-colored leather shoes, stands beneath the ethereal backdrop. It is a moment of perfection. I hold my father's arm for support as my legs labor to carry me up the gentle incline of the hill. I think how strange life is that my seventy-eight-year-old father needs to support me.

And how strange that I have never before been to see the cherry blossoms in High Park, though I have spent most of my life in Toronto. Next year I will come back to see the cherry blossoms. And I'll think of Raziel, who will never see them again. His cancer has metastasized. He is dying. His journey is coming to an end.

Finally I am a member of a club. I never wanted to belong, but now that I do, my deepest yearning is to restrict membership, to keep others out. I want to wear a T-shirt inscribed with the words *Cancer Club – Not Accepting New Members*.

14

Good Enough

TWO AND A HALF YEARS AGO my friend Claudia received the miraculous diagnosis of breast cancer, at the age of thirty-six. It was a miracle only because her diagnosis was delivered by serendipity. Collapsing in pain while watching a movie at home one night, it turned out that she had a benign ovarian cyst that had burst, which led to a slew of gynecological tests. One of the tests was a mammogram, not generally or routinely done on women of her age. Further, the tests revealed she had stage II estrogen-negative, HER2-positive breast cancer. Claudia had a lumpectomy (clean margins), a sentinel node dissection (positive pathology), an axillary node dissection (3 out of 11 nodes positive), six months of chemotherapy, six weeks of radiation therapy, and was randomized for a two-year clinical trial of the experimental drug Herceptin. I picked up a lot of the lingo from Claudia. I learned a lot more later on with my own diagnosis.

During Claudia's illness I spoke with her almost daily. There were days when she wasn't well enough to talk on the phone. There were days when the hectic pace of daily life didn't allow me to chat for long. But I tried at least to touch base every day. I went with Claudia to doctors' appointments and treatments. I sat with her in emergency rooms and hospital rooms. I took her to the hairdresser when her hair began to fall out and shopped with her when she was manic from her chemo steroids. At the time I believed that I had been close to the experience of breast cancer. When I got diagnosed, Claudia was one of the hardest people for me to tell.

Claudia had her fortieth birthday party two years after the end of her treatment. The party was three months after my own diagnosis, shortly after my first mastectomy and days before I was to start chemo. We were asked to bring, in lieu of gifts, anecdotes about Claudia. When the invited guests were done telling stories about our Claudia, she took her turn at rebuttal. "My friend Ruth said 'just because you have cancer, it doesn't make you a better person.'"

Everybody burst into nervous laughter and I could hear a few shocked gasps escape into the tension. Claudia and I looked at each other and winked discreetly. But inside, behind my overambitious smile, I wished that somehow it wasn't true. I wished that this journey I was on was some sort of elevation—but I knew that it wasn't.

To be fair to myself, the quote needs context. One night during a low point in Claudia's illness, we were chatting on the phone, as usual.

"I feel that people have expectations of me now that I have experienced cancer," she said.

"What sort of expectations?" I asked.

"To have a new perspective on life. Like the flowers should smell sweeter and their colors appear brighter. Like everything should taste more and better and I should appreciate life differently."

"Really," I replied.

"All I want is my old normal," she said. "I don't want to have to appreciate life any differently."

"I guess," I said, not fully understanding. As though I had a clue what she was talking about, I said, "You don't have to do or feel anything new, or different, or better. Hopefully this whole cancer thing is, in the grand scheme of things, just a blip on your screen of life. Just because you have had cancer doesn't make you a better person, or oblige you to change your perspective on life in any way."

Knowing now what I didn't know then, I stand by what I said—mostly. I can't help thinking that having cancer has changed my perspective, specifically regarding my own health. I will always worry more than I did before. A persistent cough will raise a red flag. A tenacious backache will spark suspicion. I truly hope that with time it will stop feeling like DEFCON 4 every time I get a papercut that could potentially become infected. I hope that down my road, the threat that the cancer might come back will feel like nothing more than the shadow of a leaf swaying in the breeze. All I want is my old reality, or at least my new reality minus the Ativan required to keep the bad thoughts at bay.

—

Shortly after my diagnosis, while I awaited surgery, a catalog arrived in the mail from a company that sells primarily mountain climbing equipment and outdoor gear. (I bought a winter jacket from them once, so they put me on their mailing list.) I do not climb mountains. I do not go camping.

I used to love camping. It was a totally laid-back, getaway-from-it-all scene. Sitting around the campfire, abusing mild substances and singing songs. Coming home dirty, hoarse-voiced, filthy and happy.

Then I had children.

Children are a lot of work. I love them, but they are a lot of work. And camping with children is like cutting off your own arms for fun. You leave behind all the amenities that help make having children less hard, like a washer and dryer, a fridge, a stove, easy access to running water, and at least a couple of doors that close behind you, and off you go into the wilderness. Despite the change of scenery and the effects of communion with nature, the children's needs and demands upon you, the parent, do not change at all. Nor should they. They still get hungry and need to be fed and watered. They still get dirty and need to be washed. And they still need to be occupied and entertained. The difference is that while camping, you, the parent, are the whole show on every front. You must begin by preparing for every eventuality before departure and fulfilling every need from fire to water to shelter once you arrive. To top it off, at the end of an exhausting day you get to sleep in a tent in a sleeping bag on the hard ground (and don't try to tell me that those thin little Therm-a-rest thingies are comfortable). In the morning, no matter the temperature outside, you awake, clammy and sore, as though you had spent the night trapped in a Ziploc sandwich bag that was dropped at a construction site, just to start all over again. And, before you can even get a cup of coffee in you, you have to fetch the water, build the fire, boil the water, and don't forget to feed the kids. That's when it's not raining. No, I don't go camping anymore.

But the catalog arrived, and in my state of almost catatonic anxiety and grief, it demanded nothing of me to lie on the couch and flip through the pictures. A mindless distraction. Looking at the colorful backpacks and grappling hooks, I realized that although I was at that moment face-to-face with my own, perhaps imminent, mortality, I was okay. I might have cancer, I might even be dying, but I was okay with my life. I didn't need to go mountain climbing or camping. I didn't have to face a list of regrets of things I should have, would have, could have . . . I was okay. No flowers needed smell sweeter, no colors needed appear brighter. I had chosen priorities, and even in the face of my own mortality I felt I had made good life decisions. My children, my husband, my family and friends, and community were the center of my universe. I had no need to appreciate life differently or subject myself to, say, camping with children to be fulfilled. If the pathology results were really bad, at least I knew my life had been well spent. If the pathology was good, I still had some major life issues to deal with, but still, I was okay. I didn't need to be a better person. I wasn't perfect, but I was good enough.

15

Shut Up and Say Yes

OR AS LONG AS I CAN REMEMBER, my mother has been packing up food for everybody and his or her sister, brother, cousin, mother, father and neighbor in need. "So and so had their wisdom teeth out, so I'm taking some soup." "So-and-so's mother died, so I'm taking some dinner." As she gets older, my mother is more often than not taking food to ailing prostates and people who can't remember her name. Nonetheless, she cooks it, packs it and schleps it even at seventy.

So I had a good teacher. If someone is ill or in need, you take food. Until I got sick I cooked almost every day. Tommy and I and our three growing boys have a sit-down dinner every night. Often, when I am cooking something, one of the boys will ask "Who is that for?" They sometimes seem surprised when I tell them it's just for us.

So, being an ex-caterer, cook, mother and Jew, my natural response to Claudia's illness had been to feed her and her family. I did not originate the paradigm; I just put it in place in that instance. I had cooked meals for other families in crisis on numerous occasions. My name had been put on a roster by somebody close to the family, and when it was my turn, I took a meal over. I wasn't randomly chosen, I volunteered, but so did a lot of other people.

You see, although we live in the urban center of Canada's biggest city, we have a unique little community. At least we like to believe it is unique. We know one another. Of course we know some people better than others. Some of our neighbors are friends, and some are acquaintances, but we take the time to interact with a lot of people. We hang out in the park and the schoolyard. We congregate in the street and on front porches. We chat while our kids swim at the local community center or play hockey at the arena. Much of our socializing takes place within a six-block radius of our house.

For what they cost, even in Toronto, the houses in our neighborhood are small. Most have backyards no bigger than an urban café patio. We have no garages or driveways and rely on unpredictable street parking. People who live elsewhere think we are fools, when for the same price in a slightly different location, we could get so much more house for our buck. Until my illness, my father had spent years repeating this mantra: "Just a little farther north and you could have more space." And true, we could use more space with three growing boys. But we are committed to our community for reasons like food rosters and the implicit understanding of the need to volunteer for them.

"I'm not comfortable asking people to cook for us every night," Claudia said.

"You're not asking," I said. "I am."

"It's a long time to expect other people to bring food," she said.

"It's not as though the same people will be bringing food every night. In fact, I don't plan to cook for you at all," I joked feebly. "Listen," I said, "there is nothing anyone can do to help other than bring food. Just shut up and say yes."

When it was my turn to have dinners delivered, Claudia threw my words back at me. "Shut up and say yes, Ruth!"

What could I say to that?

What I didn't realize at the time was that contrary to the need to actively "shut up," I would be rendered speechless by all that our family would receive. And speechless is in fact not merely an expression in this case. I am now faced with two quandaries, each in its way a question of etiquette.

First, I come from a funny family. My father is mostly silly. My mother has a dry sense of humor. My older brother makes his living as a comedian and comic writer. My younger brother is a published author, best known for his humorous essays and rapier wit. Even my kids have a keen understanding of humor. Before Micah was a year old he used the words "funny" or "not funny" to mean that he did or didn't like something.

As for me, I just can't keep my mouth shut. Wisecracks, one-liners, amusing anecdotes, I can't resist. And more than the pleasure of telling a good joke, or the capacity to entertain others or even the self-satisfaction of finding the "what's funny about it" in seemingly unfunny situations, it's one of the things that helps me recognize myself.

I'm not a fan of random gossip and dislike wanton nastiness, but I do believe funny often has an edge. That's usually what makes something funny. Only now that I have been the beneficiary of so much goodwill, I feel I can never again say anything even remotely unkind, which drastically reduces my capacity to be funny.

The second quandary rendering the otherwise loquacious me speechless is the problem of giving thanks. How does one thank so many people for so much—a plethora of goodwill, kindness, food and gifts that merits so much more than just gracious good manners. When I express my thanks on an individual, rather random basis, my sentiments are met with the usual "oh, no, it was nothing" or "it's my pleasure" and "it's the least I can do." I know these words are said with sincerity. I have not for a second felt that anybody who has reached out in any way has done so out of any sense of obligation or with any ulterior motives. While a thank you is always appreciated, I do believe that no one expects it.

So I did—I shut up and said yes. Yes to meals for my family. Yes to offers of visits or outings. Yes to books and magazines and gifts, both consumable and not. Yes to all the love and support I, we, so desperately needed to get us through. And yes to every medical intervention that was offered, no matter how brutal. But there's only so long I can be quietly accepting and grateful. I am not by nature subdued or compliant. At some point there will need to be a return to some semblance of normal, at which time I will definitely need to expand my vocabulary.

16

Layers

A FEW TIMES IN MY LIFE, I believe, I have seen myself as others must see me. Crystalline vision without the veil of self-criticism. A momentary and unexpected glimpse as I pass by a mirror in a public place, or spot myself in a photograph I don't recall having been taken. On these rare occasions, I have been surprised both by my own image and the clarity of my perception.

Returning from Thailand, at the tail end of our seven-month romp in the Far East, I wandered around the Vancouver airport awaiting my connecting flight to Los Angeles. Having been in transit for thirty-six hours, I was trying to stay awake so as not to miss the boarding call. In my travel-weary daze I watched the people in the terminal, stopping briefly to stare at a small, dark-skinned girl with long dark hair past her bum. She looked out of place amidst the mass of white faces. It took only seconds for me to realize that I was looking in a mirror. But in those few seconds, I had seen myself objectively. I was not, as I had believed for many years, a big person. I was not unattractive. And I was not, in any conventional sense, white. But the moment was fleeting, and for the most part, the impression didn't last. How I see myself has little to do with what I actually look like. Even my self-perceptive epiphany was a vision clouded by comparisons. I did not fit the conventional North American standard.

Besieged, as we are in our lives, by images of youth and beauty, it is rare to escape unscarred. In the public bathroom of the Taj Hotel, where I had taken refuge from the reality that is India on my first night in Bombay, I saw wealthy women in their multicolored saris and their lung-crushing, tight blouses as they adjusted their draperies to expose maximum rolls of blubbery opulence. Being thin in India, as I was to discover firsthand after months of intestinal disquietude, is easy. Fat is a luxury few can afford, and even fewer can sustain. But in the world in which I grew up, thin is akin to virtue. After our travels in the Far East, which included a stint in a New Delhi hospital, I returned to North America at my pre-pubertal weight, and thought I looked terrific. So did everybody else.

I have never devoted much time or effort to preening. I have actively scorned and protested the objectification of women in advertising, fashion and media. I have harassed friends with daughters for keeping *Vogue* magazines in their bathrooms, or for suggesting their girls should watch their weight. But I admit I'm not immune to the power of the images that have surrounded me throughout my life.

The year I turned forty, I decided to finally accept, and even embrace, my body. I didn't try to fool myself into loving the features that had tormented me to greater or lesser extents over the years. I simply, consciously, adopted an attitude of resigned acceptance. I would never be tall, or have long, thin legs, or a small, tight butt, or a flat stomach. Nor would I be petite and athletic looking. I would remain short and Rubenesque. No hard edges or sharp angles, but a gentle rounding and softening of surfaces would be my lot.

My decision was in small part a response to my mild emotional trepidation about my impending birthday, and to a larger extent, a logical conclusion. After looking through some old photo albums, I realized things weren't getting any better. All those pictures of me in my twenties, when I thought I was too fat, too tired, too ugly to be photographed, didn't look so bad in hindsight. In fact, the pictures only showed that with the passage of time, three pregnancies, gravity and other forces of nature, I was aging. Not prematurely, or in a frightening way, but realistically and appropriately aging. Time stands still for no man—or woman—and that included me. Thus, I concluded, inevitably I would be fatter, and rounder, and uglier in the future, and I had best accept the status quo, before the distance between my breasts and knees got any shorter, or the question "Is that a wrinkle or a shadow on the picture?" became rhetorical.

So, as the days leading to my birthday passed with ever-greater rapidity, and the weight of embarking on a new decade sat heavily upon me, I confronted one of my least attractive traits: my attitude. I would stop lamenting what I would never be, and celebrate what I was still lucky enough to have. Long live curves and cleavage! I discarded the loose-flowing robes, baggy T-shirts and oversized jeans of my youth and put what the good Lord gave me on display. Fitted jeans, tighter tops, lower necklines, and shorter skirts started to make their way into my wardrobe. It took a little time and a good deal of internal coaxing to try on the smaller size, or the more daring style, but by the time summer rolled around, I was wearing a bikini at the beach and I'd even had my belly button pierced. For the first time since I was conscious of my body having an esthetic aspect, I felt comfortable in my skin, and was happy to expose some of it.

I wasn't prancing around in clothes befitting an attention-seeking teenager or hooker (the difference being subtle at best). It's even possible that no one else noticed a difference in how I was dressing. I, on the other hand, was aware of having taken great strides. A significant paradigm shift of self-acceptance had, through no small amount of mental, motivational acrobatics, taken place. I was fabulous at forty. At least, I was more fabulous than I would no doubt be at fifty and less so than I had been at twenty. To hell with the tall, thin, fair-skinned, blonde-haired, blue-eyed images that abounded. I was confident enough, and strong enough, to love a different reality. My own. So, all things considered, I figured I would catch the wave before it crashed on the shore.

What I hadn't anticipated was that the crash would be so soon or so hard. What no one could have convinced me of, despite my new outlook, was that only a few years in the future I would grieve the loss of the body I had worked so hard to accept. I would grieve the loss of the fortitude to gracefully accept what fate had dealt me. I would grieve the loss of my immortality.

My travels in cancer-land stripped away the hard-won body confidence that I had built up layer by layer like battle armor accumulated through time and experience.

It was as if some grand, cosmic striptease had been inflicted on my mind, body and soul, leaving me beaten and vulnerable on my own stage of life.

I stand naked in front of the mirror, searching for myself where I once was. In my place stands a small, weak creature, bald from head to toe. There is no vitality in the sunken, teary eyes. No brows or lashes to protect or camouflage the fear and fragility left behind. The face is long and thin and angular, prematurely aged and lined. The complexion a mottled tone of pale green, exaggerated by the expanse of bald scalp. The shoulders are pointy and exposed. Skin pulls on the caverns created where muscle once clung to collarbones, below which a small scar runs horizontally over a small protuberance, the access point for the soul-destroying toxins. The arms hang weakly, no visible biceps or triceps to guard the bones that ache beneath the dry sheath of skin. The skeletal hands, with their brittle, bruised fingernails, appear too large on the diminished wrists that hold them.

The fingers and palms prickle with neuropathic pain, and crave to not touch, or be touched. They reach up to the purple scar tracing its path from armpit to sternum, the skin loose against the newly visible ribs. Beside the concavity of the mutilated chest, one large, pendulous, mocking breast exaggerates the absence the amputation has left. It appears out of place on this shrunken, hairless body. Not the body of a strong woman, but of a powerless child. This being has been peeled down to the barest essentials of survival, infantilized by cancer and its cures.

The mind of this stranger is fogged and slow. It holds no information, no memory, but aches for the oblivion of drugged somnolence, where it feels less pain, less sickness. The nose detects only the smells of vile chemicals that seem to emanate from every pore and orifice of this shell. The tongue cannot taste sweet or salty, only sour and bitter. The teeth hum with the sensitivity of raw nerves. The throat, the esophagus, the stomach, the bowel all burn, excoriated by the poisons that have been delivered through the veins.

The legs, with their aching bones, and the heightened sensitivity in the feet are another reminder that this body has nowhere to go. Only hospitals and doctors' appointments await, while the world goes about its business somewhere else.

Still in the company of the looking glass, I dress the body in layers to hide what is missing. I do not feel like flaunting the thinness that I have coveted in the past. It smacks of illness, of weakness, of disempowerment. I drape myself with oversized clothes, scarves and shawls. I cover my head with a hat. I paint my face. Makeup to disguise the unseemly pallor, eyelashes and eyebrows penciled in, and a rose-tinted blush on what used to be the apples of my cheeks. I do not believe anybody is fooled. The layers are gone. I am bare.

I look in the mirror and weep. I yearn to look and feel like the woman in the old photographs. The woman whose image so irked me I needed painstakingly to work up to acceptance.

I venture out into the world only as far as absolutely necessary. I cannot cope with people I do not know. I cannot play at social niceties. I am too exposed, too sensitive. Friends and family coddle me, and lie to me, saying I look terrific. I am too self-involved at this moment in my life to believe them. My self-awareness is heightened by the peeled-away layers. My world has shrunk to the size of me. I know what I look like. I do not need to happen upon myself in a mirror or photograph. There is no secret inner strength or beauty to be revealed. My outside betrays my inside. My inside betrays my outside. I see both clearly through thin skin, through rheumy eyes, through evaporated soul. I am almost dead.

—

It is gradual, but slowly, as the earth begins its spring awakening, I start to see signs of my own rebirth. The layers are returning in a variety of new and unrecognizable permutations. My hair begins growing in soft, downy tufts, almost transparent at first. Later, it thickens, darkens, and curls tighter than ever before. I develop a Jewfro in need of taming with pomades and products that have sat untouched in my bathroom for many months. By the time the weather is warm enough for bare legs and bathing suits, I am in need of waxing. (More proof that cancer is not a just mistress.) My eyelashes return as though they had never left, but my eyebrows regrow sparser than before. I read an article in the Style section of the newspaper about delicate, overgroomed brows being passé. The new fashion is bushy and bold, wouldn't you know. Maybe my brows will catch up with the trend. Maybe not. I still have my pencil.

The doctors give the go-ahead, agreeing that I am well enough to undergo another surgery—the prophylactic mastectomy of my left, healthy breast and the first stage of bilateral breast reconstruction. I walk myself to the operating room a very different person than the one who took these same steps only eight months earlier. I shed no tears.

I lie in my hospital bed feeling the effects of the anesthetic dissipating. It is late at night and I am hungry. For the first time in months, I am actually hungry. The nurse brings me food from a party they are having. I devour the sandwiches, the fruit and the tarts that she gives me. I eat so much I feel sick. I will have to learn to take it slowly.

When I return home after two nights in hospital, unlike last time, I am eager to examine myself in the mirror. The tissue expanders that have been placed in my chest under my pectoral muscles cover the concave potholes left by the mastectomies. The deflated balloons covered by muscle are in turn covered by a layer of skin that will be stretched to accommodate breast implants. For now, I am flat-chested, but with clothes on, I do not appear deformed or mutilated. *Flatsy, Flatsy, Ruth's flat and that's that*—for now. My breast surgeon comments that in a short time, my plastic surgeon will perform his magic and ta-da, "You will be restored to the barmaid you once were." I am struck that without large breasts I appear petite, and ruminate on the fact that most of the women I know who one would consider petite or small-boned are also flat-chested. It has never occurred to me before that there is a correlation between the two.

I've chosen not to use prosthetic breasts to mask my new reality. Everyone will watch my second puberty as I go through the process of expansion. Every other week, for a period of several months, I go to the breast center, where my balloons are each injected with 50 cc's of saline solution. It does not hurt, but it does feel strange. They advise me to get some patterned shirts to help camouflage

the irregular shapes sometimes encountered through the
. inflation process. I have always worn solid colors, and
feel overwhelmed by the idea of introducing a new style
choice into my wardrobe right now. I compromise and
buy two tank tops with pictures on them—one Wonder
Woman, one Curious George—that match my early adolescent body.

I think about photographing myself through the
stages of my rebirth and wonder who would ever be
interested. Friends of ours have a beautiful series of
pictures of their first child as a newborn taken beside
different pieces of fruit. The photos are sequential,
taken at one-week intervals until the baby was six weeks
old, and thereafter monthly, until her first birthday. In
each photo, the baby lies next to a different piece of
fruit, which provides perspective regarding her size
and growth. I think about embarking on a project of
this sort and decide that breakfast food would provide
the most appropriate juxtaposition. First I could pose
beside a pair of pancakes, then perhaps some thick-
cut toast, English muffins, fried eggs, half grapefruits.
I decide that while some might see the humor in it, I am
not brave enough to record what is still a trying ordeal.
I settle for letting anybody who is curious feel my breast
mounds. I cannot feel anything anyhow, and it's not like
they are real.

The mind fog and depression that were a by-product of the chemo drugs begins to lift. I get some assistance from an antidepressant prescribed to help alleviate the overwhelming hot flashes brought on by my drug-induced menopause. (My doctors say I will have to take medication to block any estrogen in my body from feeding cancer growth for at least five years.) I can see glimmers of my personality returning and manage to find humor in the dichotomy of going through puberty and menopause all at the same time.

I ache to create something. I need to do so to feel normal. The neuropathy in my hands, another side effect from chemotherapy, prevents me from pursuing anything sculptural, my preferred form of creativity, so I turn to writing, and find both refuge and salvation through fountain pen and notebooks.

My hunger returns with a vengeance and my taste buds rejoice in flavors they had forgotten. I have no time or patience for entertainment that does not include food. The little energy and strength that has returned is directed toward grocery shopping, cooking and eating. Over three short months I regain the twenty-five pounds I lost. None of it is muscle. I feel fat and bloated as I re-don my pre-cancer clothes. I am not comfortable. I am not strong. I do not fit into my old mold.

I have replaced my amputated breasts with two

brand-new ones, complete with artificial nipples and areolae. And though the new breasts are high and firm, and I am grateful to my wonderful plastic surgeon for giving them to me, I miss my old breasts. I miss being able to feel when they are touched. I am self-conscious of them not matching the rest of my middle-aged body. I wonder if it is just a matter of time before they feel like they are actual breasts, as opposed to reasonable facsimiles of breasts. I wonder if I will eventually be able to assume ownership of them, rather than thinking of them as being a bit like strap-on novelty boobies. With luck, by the time my energy and confidence return to meet my new hair and new breasts, I will have found the necessary strength required to love my old ass and thighs.

17

Waste Not, Want Not

I AM A COLLECTOR. I collect things of beauty, things of potential use, things of personal historical significance or memory, clothes, shoes, and miscellaneous stuff. I do not haunt secondhand stores or yard sales looking for treasures to add to my collections. I acquire things in a less directed, organic sort of way. It is only through conscious introspection that I am even aware of my propensity to hang on to things others might discard without a second thought, or lose and replace dozens of times seasonally, annually, in a lifetime.

It feels a little like a confession of a dingy secret—too benign to be dark or truly dirty—but perhaps a quirkiness that might over time turn me into the kind of old woman who is referred to, behind her back of course, as eccentric.

Some of my collecting is simple lack of attrition and an almost panicky reaction to waste, no doubt inherited from my mother. I do not lose the things most people misplace regularly—hats, gloves, scarves, swim goggles, glasses, keys, earrings. I have them all. The ski mittens I have been wearing since ninth grade, now shabby and threadbare, I still wear to play with my kids each winter. The first pair of dangly earrings that I bought at age twelve with my own money and eagerly put into my newly pierced ears, a little too soon before the fresh wounds had completely healed. My embroidery hoops and thread, which I used to embellish my many pairs of Lee jeans. Seashells and smooth sand-beaten bits of varied colored glass, which I have gathered on beaches around the world and squirreled away in backpacks, suitcases and duffel bags, each one a reminder of a specific stroll on a particular stretch of sand marking my passage through time. Beads, stickers, watches—I have them all.

When something breaks or wears out, I replace it only reluctantly. Not because of any particular attachment to the thing itself, or as an affectation of some minimalist ideal. I have lots of stuff. I suppose the need to replace socks or gloves because they have worn thin evokes in me a mild sense of disappointment that nothing lasts forever. Even then, most things get "purposed down." Old bandanas become everyday napkins, become kids' costume-box accessories, become art and craft supplies, become dust rags and so on.

During a family visit to South Africa when I was seven, we stopped over in Rio de Janeiro for a few days. As we sat on a veranda at the back of our hotel across the road from Copacabana Beach, a waiter appeared with a large platter full of fruit the likes of which I had never seen. Deep purple, sweet figs, with syrupy crunchy insides that made the dried figs I had eaten at home stuffed in Fig Newton cookies seem pathetic. Mangoes and papayas and lychees, watermelon and pineapple, all of it fragrant and enticing. It was a life-altering moment.

While we were in Rio, my parents bought me a pair of white leather sandals. To this day, just as the Brazilian fruit is the standard by which I measure all fruit, those sandals represent for me the zenith of sandals. There was the softness of the supple leather and the comfort of the completely flat bottom; the gently arched sole that supported my small foot in exactly the right spot between my heel and the ball—a place I hardly knew existed before I met these shoes. I remember how pretty I thought my sun-bronzed toes looked in those spanking white Brazilian sandals. When I grew out of them, it was many years before my mother could get me to wear other sandals. Some things are more difficult to replace than others.

Nonetheless, eventually my feet found comfort in other shoes. The perfectly patched favorite jeans are replaced by new, stiff denims that need work and time to feel right. The wallet with exactly the right number of compartments but a broken zipper is put aside for a new one that will one day be the one that is difficult to replace. Ultimately, they are just things. They can be replaced.

One of my favorite children's stories is about a little boy whose grandfather is a tailor. On the occasion of the boy's birth, the grandfather makes him a beautiful blanket. As the cherished blanket becomes worn, the boy's mother encourages him to throw it out. The boy insists that his grandfather can fix it, and so the old man does again and again, transforming the blanket into a jacket, then a vest, a necktie, and finally a button, which eventually pops off and rolls down a sewer grate. The boy, much older by the end of the story, grieves the final loss of his prized possession only briefly. He realizes that what he is left with is material for a wonderful story.

Wonderful stories account for further collectibles. Cards, letters and photographs are all packed away in boxes, or labeled in albums. Each package is a tangible account of different phases and stages of my life. I very much doubt that anybody else will ever care to peruse the

carefully cataloged contents of my childhood, my adolescence, my travels or my parties. Nonetheless, I have kept it
all. In fact, I fear that I will drop dead and my children will
have to go through all my stuff and ask, "Why on earth did
she keep all this crap?" Perhaps what will surprise them is
that I also kept all of their stuff. Things out of which
stories are told and memories evoked. I have, in other
carefully labeled bins, boxes and files, their school work,
art projects, birthday cards from friends and family,
homemade Mother's Day gifts and birthday treasures,
report cards, concert programs, baby teeth, locks of hair.
Oh God, as I write it all down, it does sound quite mad.

So why collect all these tokens of our fleeting lives? Not
just for the tales that might be woven, or the remembrance
of things past do I hold on to these scraps of paper or objects
of no commercial or readily discernible value. I believe
that it is immeasurably important to our human psyche to
exist within a context as opposed to a vacuum. These
things that mark our lives allow me to believe that I am not
only here and now. Something came before me, something
will come after me. Whether I leave a mark in time in any
monumental way or not, at least I can plot my own passage
through this life. Someone else can throw it away later.

What's more, cool stuff can be made into other cool
stuff. I have always made things and now my children
make things too. When, for my mother's seventieth

birthday, each of the boys undertook an elaborate art project, I was delighted to be able to produce for them from my secret stores and stashes exactly the right materials. For Micah's hand-knit purse in lime green and burnt orange hues, I provided velvet ribbon in orange and mustardy green with matching floss to appliqué onto the bag and esthetically hide the seams of his ambitious design. Out of oven-baked modeling material, Amit sculpted the yellow convertible my mother has always longed for. I delivered a piece of stiff, transparent plastic to cut into the appropriate size for the car's windshield and five perfect buttons for the headlights, taillights and steering wheel. Safi's papier-mâché self-portrait bust was crying out for hair and a suitable stand. Thank God I had saved some brown ribbon and yarn and some aluminum ductwork, which we easily secured with my handy hot-glue gun.

Who knows what disaster might have ensued when Micah arrived home with half a dozen friends needing to construct a city, infrastructure and all, for a school project, had I not hung on to bits and pieces. Old corks still with the faint fragrance of the wine they once stopped, plasticine, tubes of paint, brushes, small tins that once contained tiny mints, plastic spools no longer holding thread, felt-tip markers and lots of hot-glue sticks helped those kids secure A's in geography.

In this way, I can almost justify my idiosyncratic

WHEN MY WORLD WAS VERY SMALL

holding on to objects others blithely discard. I must, however, confess an unrelated source of collectibles. I love beautiful, shiny, colorful things, both found and purchased. Eccentric shoes and clothes in colors or styles so wild they are never either in nor out of fashion, hang in my closet for upwards of twenty years. Textiles, masks and small objects from various trips bedeck every surface. Numerous sets of dishes, serving platters, vases, and colored glass vessels fill nooks and shelves in our home. But most of all, red is my color of covet. It is not necessarily my favorite color, but when confronted by red commodities I often lack the fortitude to resist the temptation to buy.

Though these confessions might bring to mind a chaotic environment most commonly inhabited by an individual afflicted with a diagnosable psychopathology, I assure you our home is lovely. Everything has a place, and when called upon to procure the perfect thingamajig, I know exactly where to look.

While I am as guilty as anybody in our family of contributing to the clutter of a busy household, from time to time it overwhelms me and a manic purge is necessary to restore a sense of order. The rules are simple: put it away, give it away or throw it away. However, it is only I, the self-confessed collector, who gets overwhelmed by the stuff that accumulates, and therefore only I feel the urge to purge.

During the months of my illness and treatment I felt utterly defeated by the accumulation of stuff. Since everything must have a place, it was enormously frustrating not to possess the energy for putting things away. In parallel to this sense that my world was descending into both physical and metaphysical chaos, I nevertheless continued to collect. Hundreds of cards wishing me well were carefully accumulated in a happy red box purchased expressly for that purpose. Medical documents, information, schedules and appointments were all neatly organized in a portable folder. Dozens of generous gifts of scarves, shawls, pajamas, bathrobes and slippers were accumulated. Snacks of every texture and taste experience were brought to my bedroom in the hope that I might find something palatable. Articles of jewelry with magical cabalistic powers, crystals, and a necklace inscribed with the word *Believe* which was given to me anonymously by a group of women in my neighborhood. And a continuous stream of small, shiny, pretty trinkets were brought to me by my six-year-old friend Bridget, who was not quite sure what was wrong with me, but entirely convinced that her precious treasures would help the situation. All things newly introduced into our environment and waiting for their place to be determined.

To further contribute to the rapid influx of stuff, there was an entire catalog of cancer-specific items. There were two wigs, which I had bought prior to losing all my hair but was unable to wear when the time came. I tried them on on a couple of occasions and felt distinctly "Mrs. Bates." Hence, a tsunami of hats of every description came my way. Bottles of pills to remedy the horrific side-effects of chemo made my bathroom look like a well-stocked pharmacy. A post-mastectomy camisole, equipped with pockets to hold surgical drains and soft, foam breast forms. A copper wire head massager that looked like a grade school sculptural representation of a daddy long legs touted to be soothing to people going through chemo. Calendars filled with the names of people who brought us dinners for months on end according to a carefully organized schedule coordinated by my friends Cathy and Kate. Menus that accompanied some of the meals to help us navigate the numerous disposable containers of delicacies that appeared nightly. Two mastectomy bras containing pockets to hold a prosthetic breast, one black and one red (of course). And one asymmetrical right silicone breast form carefully removed nightly and placed in its form-fitting box at the bottom of my closet.

I knew I was beginning to feel better when summer rolled around and it became impossible for me to look beyond the mounting chaos. It began with an impotent yearning to restore order, one I had insufficient strength to act upon. Over days and weeks my energy slowly started to return and with it, on a Lilliputian scale, my ability to focus. The inevitable purge was approaching, and while I waited for the physical capacity to "put it away, give it away or throw it away," I fantasized about what would become of the trappings of cancer that had found their way into my life.

My children wanted the wigs for masquerade potential, and initially I agreed that when I was sure I no longer needed them they could take up residence in the costume box. But when my hair actually did begin to sprout, I just didn't want them around, those two wigs on their creepy fake heads with painted faces of overdone makeup and lips that were at the same time pouty and too small and a color that no mouth should ever be. I figured, given that wigs can be quite costly, somebody in need could certainly use them. I dropped them off at the chemo clinic in a bag with a note attached which read: *Brand new, please feel free to take.* Why I felt sheepish about it I don't yet know.

Having reneged on my promise of the wigs to the boys, I decided they could have the four soft-form breasts that I used as temporary prosthetics while my surgical wounds healed. These I also delivered without announcement or fanfare. The next time they sifted through the costume box they could decide what mythical beauty or beast required a D-cup lump or bump.

Then there were the hats, worn for months on end. The ones that were comfortable but hideous I could not in good conscience allow any cancer patient to acquire, so I did not take them to the clinic. Those I left at the thrift store. The other hats presented a dilemma. As much as I would love to have the power to prevent further member-ship in the cancer club, I don't. Sooner or later someone I know will be diagnosed, and having taken the journey myself, I might in some way be able to provide a special brand of comfort or support. At the very least I can provide some reasonable-looking headgear. I packed the hats away in a see-through plastic pouch with a zipper, saved from a long-ago purchase of a baby blanket. (I knew it would come in handy someday.)

Too soon, my stash would be called upon, when I found out that my cousin had been diagnosed with breast cancer. A plain cotton hat, a copper wire head massager, and a discreetly wrapped post-mastectomy camisole, all found a new home with my cousin. I can only hope they will be of some use to her.

The leftover antinausea meds could easily have been flushed down the toilet, but at forty dollars a pill it seemed like a terrible waste. Did I mention that I hate waste? Though I am not a medical professional, I have often and freely given medical advice, and shared prescription drugs with friends in need. These were different. I couldn't presume to take responsibility for these drugs. I gave them to a doctor who I knew would help them find their way to somebody with no drug plan.

The bras, one black, one red (of course), each with a pocket to hold a prosthesis, owe no one anything. They worked hard and provided an invaluable service. They were honorably discharged to the garbage pail. No tears were shed.

Order was being restored and my space was being exorcised. The cancer demons and their accompanying baggage were moving on. One thing remains. I cannot come up with a single appropriate destination for one asymmetrical right silicone breast prosthesis. Too grotesque for the costume box, too personal for an anonymous clinic drop-off. I have a somewhat sick curiosity that is begging me to cut it open with a knife and poke around inside it, but at four hundred dollars a tit, the waste outweighs the childish fascination. Maybe I'll sell it on eBay.

18

The Year I Cannot Taste

I DREAM THAT I AM RUNNING. I am not running fast, or far, or for a long time, but effortlessly. I am running for a bus or a light. It is unspectacular. There is no sense of accomplishment, nor any feeling of panic or stress. My legs easily adopt the pace. My arms swing freely. My body does not burden me, limit me. My subconscious mind remembers who I was.

I dream that I am cooking. I am preparing an elaborate feast. There will be a celebration and I am the host. The preparation is labor-intensive and the food ornate. The quantities are vast. It is a labor of joy and love. I am excited by the event of the preparation itself. I do not feel overwhelmed or nauseated. In my dream I hungrily taste each festive concoction and rejoice in the sensual flavors and textures. My subconscious recalls my true relationship with food, with joy, with life.

During my illness, I would dream these dreams repeatedly. The weaker I became, the more I dreamt about running. The more difficulty I was having eating, the more I dreamt about cooking. My conscious mind and body, trapped in the narcissism of illness, would be consumed by pain, anguish, loneliness and fear. But, once asleep, the color of experience seeped beyond my consciousness into my dreams, where I would remember the way things felt.

The conscious memories I hold are a series of gastro-nomic events. I remember where I've been by what I ate. I recall celebrations by what was served. The thought of a particular food can bring to mind a place, a person, a moment in time. Conversely, a place or person can stim-ulate recollection of a taste. It is an inextricable part of my whole; a mnemonic device that contextualizes every-thing in my life.

I know, for example, that my cousin's first son was born in April of 1990. I know because I was in Thailand at the time. I went to the weekend market on the outskirts of Bangkok and bought a baby gift—a tiny hill tribe outfit labeled *24 months*—which my cousin kindly squeezed her oversized four-month-old into for the occasion of our first meeting.

I remember going to the weekend open-air market because I ate something remarkable there. At one of the many food stalls I pointed at what appeared to be thinly sliced beef in a glistening, gooey sauce. The vendor ladled some ice water with jasmine flowers floating in it from a ceramic crock on the ground into a pale green porcelain bowl. Using a pair of bamboo tongs, he carefully plucked a hand-sized piece of meat from the steaming pile and dropped it into the bowl of ice water. Somewhat confused, but already committed to the transaction, I took the bowl and chopsticks that were offered and sat on a wooden crate nearby. Fishing into the icy water with the sticks, I extracted the crystallized meat, catching jasmine blossoms clinging to the adhesive shell that had formed. Raising my hand above my head, I dangled the large piece of meat into my mouth, and bit through the crackly, honey-syrup crust into the salty, tender meat, while jasmine flowers melted on my tongue. It was unlike anything I had ever experienced before. When I think about it, I don't just get the taste and the texture of the beef, I get the whole market, all of my purchases, the weather, and even the shoes I was wearing.

I have many cousins, and they have many children. I cannot claim to remember when each of them was born—unless I ate something noteworthy at the time.

I like to take hypothetical walks through my life, recalling what I ate where, and see what other memories are evoked in the process. If, for example, I start with eating passion fruit ice-lollies on Muizemberg Beach in Cape Town, I can reconstruct vast portions of our family trip to South Africa when I was seven years old. I can remember the euphoria of playing putt-putt near the beach with a large gaggle of newly met cousins. In the distant recesses of my mind, I can hear my mother's South African accent intensifying as she easily readopts the local lilts in conversation with numerous unknown adults who insist that I call them "Auntie" or "Uncle." I blush when I think of my brothers entertaining everybody from the top of a picnic table at an engagement party with show tunes from the movie *Oliver!* The smell of the sea. The wind on the beach. The hairpin turns on mountain roads. My mother's lime green two-piece suit—was it pants or a skirt? And, in my mind's eye I clench my teeth together to crunch down on the small black seeds encased in the sweet fruity ice of the frozen passion fruit treat.

Through gastronomic recollection, I can travel through time and relive or re-experience events and reacquaint with people. A single dish gives access to endless memories. For example, take chicken soup with matzo balls. My mother's light, fluffy matzo balls. My mother-in-law's denser, saltier matzo balls. Realizing when I served my friend Angela matzo balls that they are only comfort food if you grew up on them. Auntie Lorna's baked matzo balls with fried onions, or cinnamon and raisins. Passover in New York with the Long Island cousins. Passover in Montreal with the Dunskys. Lilliane's hard-boiled egg and saltwater soup. Hard-boiled egg separated and grated into yellow and white Stars of David, on platters of chopped liver or chopped herring, by Blumé. Chopped herring with kichlach. Auntie Riva's kichlach. My grandmother's kichlach and taiglach, hidden in the kitchen bench in Montreal. She visited and baked when I was only four or five years old. Yet, through the miracle of food recall, I can remember.

I can use my food memory for quick reference about time and place by playing "the best" game. Try it. Think of a food and remember where and when you ate the best example of that food. You can even set stricter parameters, for example, types of fruit.

THE BEST FRUIT

    Mandarin oranges – *Luxor, November 1989*

    Strawberries – *Local, Ontario, every June*

    Blueberries, Wild – *Quebec City, August 2001*

    Figs – *Rio de Janeiro, December 1969*

    Mangoes – *Bangkok, April 1990*

But the quick reference triggers a memory and makes my nostrils flare, searching the air for ghosts of fragrant delights long past. It is the middle of the night, and Tommy and I are making our way through the hot, humid air of Bangkok streets in search of the flower market. There, all the flowers from around the countryside are delivered for distribution locally and for export. On our way, we pass a street stall selling great mounds of perfectly ripe, small, golden mangoes, their perfume so sweet it is like a drug. We hand the vendor the equivalent of about twenty-five cents and he fills a crinkly, cellophane shopping bag with the fruit.

We make our way toward the flower market, which we smell before we can see it. The heady aroma of orchids wafts through the thick night air. Suddenly, we are standing in the middle of mountains and mountains of fresh orchids in shades of pink and purple and yellow and white. The sweat runs down our bodies, and the bodies of the endless tiny, sinewy men unloading truckloads of flowers into voluminous piles. The musky smell of body odour intermingling with the perfume of the endless orchids is intoxicating. We fish mangoes from the bag hanging on my wrist and, using our teeth and fingers, peel back the leathery skin, revealing the slippery, golden flesh. I bite into my fruit and the sweet pulp splashes against my cheeks and tongue and slithers down my throat. Sticky mango juice runs down my chin onto my neck and rivulets of golden nectar wind their way from my fingers down my arms, pooling in the crevices at my elbows, mixing with my sweat. I stand watching the hive of market activity buzz and hum while I eat one succulent mango after another, not stopping to mop up. My senses are on fire. I am ecstatically happy. I will never forget this moment or these mangoes.

When we were children my mother occasionally would take my two brothers and me to Yorkdale shopping mall for dinner. As a full-time working physician, she had little time for errands or shopping. I suppose that if she needed to buy something, the evening was her only opportunity. She would give each of us a dollar or two, and leave us to buy our own dinner while she went to shop. The three of us would make our way to a fried chicken place at one end of the mall near the supermarket. Pooling our resources, we would carefully work out what to buy, what to share, and what would be for personal consumption. With some combination of greasy fried chicken, onion rings and Coca-Cola slushies (served with plastic straws splayed at one end to create a spoon-like feature), the three of us would sit together on the high chrome stools at the chicken counter devouring our fatty feast. I felt independent and empowered beyond belief.

It is not uncommon for me to go out of my way to procure a particular treat, or to plan an adventure or travel route because there is something I want to eat in a particular direction. Detours through Montreal en route to or from the Laurentian Mountains or the Eastern Townships for Schwartz's smoked meat. Late-night walks to East Jerusalem for *sachleb*—a sweet, thin, milky pudding made from orchids, served hot and garnished with pistachios and pine nuts. From a large samovar on a wheeled cart, the Arab vendor would dispense his edible perfume into brittle, disposable plastic cups that warmed our hands as we walked back to the Jewish neighborhoods through the cool night. But, alas, that was in the old days, when it was still relatively safe to wander into East Jerusalem late at night. It is not only the *sachleb* I recall, it is an entire political era.

And there are things I eat not because I particularly like them, or even necessarily want them, but because they are an intrinsic part of my food-time-memory-recall continuum. Skating on the Rideau Canal in Ottawa demands that I eat a sweet, greasy, flat donut sprinkled with cinnamon, sugar and lemon juice, known locally as a Beaver Tail. A birthday party is not a birthday party without Cheezies. One can not be in New York City without eating a hot pretzel slathered in yellow mustard from a street vendor. How would you even know you had been to Jaffa unless you stopped at Abulafia for a fresh-baked pita covered in peppery, fried onions and a sunny-side-up egg with a broken yolk, hot from the giant ovens that face the street?

—

My gobsmackingly surprising response to being diagnosed with cancer, was that I lost my appetite. My nervous stomach, compounded by the side effects of surgery, anesthetics and months of chemotherapy, resulted in my eating minimally for the better part of a year. The strange fallout is that without the benefit of having tasted much of anything for those many months, I cannot remember things that would under normal circumstances be added to the virtual pages of my personal life history and experience. I seem to have lost a year of my life.

Oddly, the year I cannot taste, the one I therefore cannot remember, is the one about which I have written, and written, and written, amassing many notebooks full of experiences and recollections. In my desperation to emerge healthy and whole from my journey in cancer I have dug deeper inside myself than ever before. But I wonder: Without taste to attach to memory do I simply have to accept that that is time lost forever? Can I reclaim any of it?

A friend once told me that nothing he ever did in his whole life was good enough or bad enough to impress his father.

His father's measuring tape, the thing against which everything else was juxtaposed, was Auschwitz. His experiences in the Holocaust defined his entire life, and his perceptions of the lives of everyone he encountered.

"You think that's bad? Feh! That's nothing."

"You don't know from hungry."

"You don't know from tired."

"This? This is what you call hard work?"

This, this is what I call "Baseline Auschwitz." Of course everything else pales in comparison. There can be no greater suffering. And joy, and happiness, and rejoicing, and celebration, also trumped by liberation of the camps, reunification with siblings presumed murdered, survival. How can a graduation, a bar mitzvah, a wedding compare? It can't.

I do not want to live the rest of my life with "Baseline Cancer." I do not want this brief but intense period of my life to be the experience against which all else is measured. I must coax other experiences back to the surface, where they can suppress Baseline Cancer and keep it from taking over.

I cannot, however, escape the reality that our experiences shape us. So, how can I best use this experience of which I can only remember the crisis, the suffering, and that which is self-referential? As in my dreams, I can try to remember the way things felt. I can glean from the experiences of others where my memory is vague. Perhaps I can excavate some positive aspects of my missing year and retroactively attach flavors to things worth remembering from my previous taste lexicon.

I can remember the feeling of Tommy's love and devotion in his selfless caring for me and the children. I can try to emulate his unyielding efforts to fill in the gaps left by my temporary abdication of duties, and maintenance of order and sanity in a time of disorder and insanity. Perhaps these might best be recalled as the depth of the deepest darkest chocolate.

I can learn from my mother, Gina, that the role of a parent is never done. I can remember how important it was to have her with me at all my appointments and procedures. That there are times when sitting quietly by is more important than offering up any words. That there are times when a hand to hold is more important than anything. Benign and dependable like scrambled eggs on toast.

I can be grateful for the love of my sons and thankful for everything they did to help, and every meltdown they had, to remind me that not everything is about me. Something spicy to call attention to my tongue and remind me that it is how the outside world comes in and how my inside communicates with the outside.

I can cherish the support of my father and my brothers and the remarkable relationships they have with my husband and children, their generosity of time and spirit. Chinese food ordered to be shared among everyone at the table.

I can draw upon the examples of unfaltering and unconditional friendship set by my many friends. I can be encouraged by all my fellow travelers who have moved past Baseline Cancer. I can be inspired by the unflinching hospitality shown to my children by so many friends. I can be humbled by the selflessness of all those who provided us with generous meals. Large salads, varied and colorful and necessary for health and well-being.

I can recall the dozens of bouquets of flowers that were sent by friends and family, both near and far. The endless parade of visitors who didn't allow me to fall so deep into my rabbit hole that the climb out was impossible. Carrots?

19

Just Keep Swimming

Most of my life I have been a swimmer. As a child, there were entire days I spent in the water, inventing games of a varied, theatrical or athletic nature. Who can swim the farthest under water? Who can do the fanciest dive? Who's the fastest? Who can do the best impression of a drunk walking off a diving board? Or, without the luxury of company, there was the meditative repetition of allowing myself to sink deep in the water, exhaling bubbles slowly, till my lungs were empty. The lattice-like reflections of the sun on the dappled water gently undulating on the pale blue pool bottom. My vertical body floating back to the surface only long enough to refill the sacks inside my chest with new air and then descending again into the deep. Over and over like a mantra till I was overcome with peace and relaxation. Getting out of the water only to lie like a sea lion on the sun-warmed concrete. Water seemed a part of my natural habitat.

In my final year of high school, we had a year-long physiology project that required us to run at least four times a week for twenty minutes and graph our progress by measuring heart rate before and after each run and showing the distance covered. It was a thinly disguised attempt by the physiology teacher, who also happened to be the gym teacher, to force a bunch of lazy teenagers to be physically active. Not a bad idea, and since it counted for a large percentage of our final grade, which many of us needed for university applications, we complied. When I developed shin splints from running without warming up, (which would have required extra effort) my teacher suggested that I try to complete my graphs by swimming instead of running. That's when I discovered two things. First, that it is much easier to elevate one's heart rate by running than by swimming. Second, that I was a really strong swimmer. I had known I was confident in the water, but it wasn't until then that I realized I could comfortably swim *forever* without getting tired. I wasn't fast, but I was consistent, and for me, compared with running, swimming seemed effortless.

When I got to university, the endless hours of sitting and reading needed to be balanced by some physical activity. I did not come to this conclusion because of a natural inclination to exercise, but through shock therapy: the terrible shock when I stepped on a scale at the end of my first semester and realized I'd best get off my ass before it grew so big it needed to pay separate tuition. I began to swim daily at the University Athletic Centre, steeling myself against the insecurities aroused by the presence of *truly* athletic students. I imagined myself in a chrysalis as I walked down the long, frigid corridor, past the weight room to the pool. It did not matter who else was there. I was alone. As I dove in, the water engulfed me, cleansed me, renewed me. I swam. An hour. A hundred laps. A mile.

I continued to swim, almost religiously, save for a few gaps during periods of my life when I didn't have access to a pool. I don't particularly enjoy it, but I recognize that it contributes to a better quality of life for me. If I were the kind of person who fell asleep easily at night, perhaps I wouldn't swim. If I did not suffer from joint pain, perhaps I wouldn't swim. If I could manage to clear my mind in any other way, perhaps I wouldn't swim. But I do not, and I do, and I can't, so I swim. And when I swim, I do and I don't and I can.

For the past nine years I have been swimming at the Boys' and Girls' Club community center around the corner from my house. I like swimming there more than at almost any pool I have frequented over the years. I am comfortable with the warmth of the water, kept at a steamy 92 degrees Fahrenheit for the sake of the young children who take lessons there. I am at ease with the proletarian nature of the facilities—pool, change room, shower room—no lockers or saunas or frills.

Despite the utilitarian character of "my" pool it has taken on some of the attributes people no doubt seek out in exclusive, private clubs. It is almost never crowded during the morning lap swim that I attend. There is usually an influx of newbies immediately following the Christmas break—people trying to fulfill New Year's resolutions pertaining to health and fitness. But by mid-January the pool empties out and only the regulars are left. The regulars are a group of fewer than a dozen middle-aged women like myself. (Perhaps they would take offense to being referred to as middle-aged, but given the alternative I would personally consider myself lucky if this does, in fact, turn out to be my middle age.) Nobody among us is fanatically fit, or driven to swim. Everybody swims at her own pace, in her own space, on her own schedule. We are not joiners. We are not competitors. We need no one else's approval or cajoling. We swim. Though we swim alone, we are comforted by one another's consistent presence. And then, in the shower, we do not feel ashamed of our time-thickened waistlines, our gravity-slung breasts, our stretch-mark-stained bellies. Through running water and shampoo suds, we talk about art and literature. As we towel off, we converse about education, health care, movies. We cream our chlorine-crusted skin and clothe ourselves through interesting chat. We are un-members of a silent un-sisterhood of swimmers.

Before my children were sophisticated enough for serious adult movies, I took them to any children's movie that was in the theaters. Some were dreadful, and even painful to endure, others moderately diverting. Occasionally a children's movie managed to both entertain and inspire me, because of either its inventiveness or its production quality. And always appreciated were elements of plot or humor purposely pitched at the adults in the audience. For instance, in *Finding Nemo*, the subplot about parental worries vis-à-vis their children was what kept me going. It was, however, one fleeting moment in this particular movie that I ended up adopting as a personal philosophy. The comic-relief clownfish character, Dory, who can't retain a thought longer than, well, a fish, gets confused repeatedly about what it was she was in the middle of doing, and consoles herself with the repeated singsong "Just keep swimming, just keep swimming . . ." It seemed to me an apt notion. No matter what happens, no matter what gets in the way, no matter what life throws at you, just keep swimming.

I had planned to continue swimming through my cancer treatments. I had my mother sew a pocket into one of my bathing suits to hold my prosthetic breast. I opted for a Port-A-Cath instead of a PICC line for chemotherapy. In my mind I played out scenarios of how I would change and shower without revealing my amputation, saving myself and others from awkwardness. I thought about getting a Lycra bathing cap for when I lost my hair. At one point I mentioned to my father that I was feeling self-conscious about putting on a bathing suit and he suggested I simply wear a T-shirt over my bathing suit. Ah ya, I thought—the wet T-shirt—that age-old bastion of female modesty.

But six weeks after surgery I began chemotherapy, and with the first round I was so wiped out that I stopped imagining I could go to the pool. My theoretical solutions seemed to have no bearing on reality. The pool, still just two blocks from home, seemed too far away; the water, still 92 degrees Fahrenheit, too cold to enter. I could not "just keep swimming." I was too busy drowning.

Just over a year after my diagnosis, with chemotherapy and two surgeries behind me, I need to start building up the strength I have lost. I am not the me I used to be. I need cajoling. I need approval. I join my friends Kate and Jane on their daily morning walks. They are kind and humor me, slowing their pace so I can keep up. Jane holds my hand and pulls me up or waits for me at the top of stairs. She cheers me on, swearing she can see a radiance emanating from within me as I labor to climb. I'm sure it is just the sweat that flows with my effort. Jane becomes my personal trainer, motivational speaker and Sherpa all rolled into one. At times she practically carries me up modest inclines that feel like the foothills of the Himalayas.

When she has bolstered me with enough encouragement and protected me with enough spiritual and physical strength, feeling the chill of winter in the air, it is time to return to "my" pool. Embarrassed by my drastically deteriorated strength (in some illogical way I feel this is an indication of personal failure) I choose to go swimming at midday, avoiding the morning regulars. It is not a rational decision. The morning swimmers are my friends. They have seen me and supported me through all the ordeals of the past year. But I am tired of being weak and needy. I want people to see the old me—perhaps then I too will be able to see her.

I swim slowly. Slower than I ever have. My back aches as my arms pull themselves through the water, awakening dormant muscles I had forgotten existed. The water feels viscous and heavy around my stiffened joints, my atrophied strength. But I persevere. I must climb out of this hole. I must swim back to health. This is not a choice. I must move forward.

After several weeks of swimming at midday, I call Cathy and ask her if she wants to swim with me in the morning. I know she will be there anyhow, but I have a need to cushion my reentry. I am announcing my intention to rejoin the un-group. I arrive at the community center and am greeted warmly in the dressing room. I feel a collective sigh, an exhaling of held breath on my behalf. We have all come out on the other side.

In the pool there is a sense of celebration. The prodigal has returned. Cathy queries the appropriateness of early morning champagne. The event of my return is significant not just to me.

I swim. I swim. I swim.

I am struck by a thought as I swim with three other women. I am struck by the thought that all these women have endured significant crises in their lives. One lost a sister to lung cancer only a few years ago. *Just keep swimming.* Two have special needs children who will require significant care and support their whole lives. *Just keep swimming.* One had two children with cancer. *Just keep swimming.* One of those two children died from her leukemia. *Just keep swimming.*

I am also struck by the thought that though I am swimming and I am strengthening my body and emptying my mind, I am thinking. I am thinking about other people's problems, not only about myself. I can feel my world getting bigger. And if I just keep swimming, maybe I will find my way into rivers and lakes and oceans till my world can once again be the size of the world.

ACKNOWLEDGMENTS

The Marathon

MY FRIEND ANNIE has told me that at certain points in a twenty-six-mile run one is more susceptible to losing focus, stamina, hope, strength or whatever it is one needs to sustain the will and drive to finish a marathon. (Though it is beyond me where one finds the will to begin the marathon in the first place.) At these points, friends come and run along with her for a portion of the distance.

No one who joins Annie claims to have run the race for her. It is Annie's marathon. Like fighting cancer, no one can do it for you. They can't even walk in your shoes. (You need your shoes to stay in the race.) But they can run shorter stretches alongside you and help give you the strength you might lack on your own to stay the course.

A few years ago, Vanessa, a woman from our neighborhood, was hit by a truck. Both of her arms were broken. She was lucky that she suffered only broken arms, everybody said. Lucky or not, she still needed to eat. So, of course, we cooked for her and her family. Secretly, to ourselves, we said a silent *There but for the grace of God go I.* Even the nonbelievers and skeptics among us.

About a year later, Vanessa was found by her husband John lying on the floor of their home in a coma. She was rushed to the hospital, where she remained comatose for several weeks. No one knew if she would survive the meningitis that had attacked her brain. Again we cooked. We cooked until, miraculously, Vanessa was able once again to cook for her own family.

Vanessa's husband John was so overwhelmingly grateful for the outpouring of community support he and his family received that he felt compelled to pay it forward in some significant way. When he heard of an acquaintance of his who needed a kidney, he offered one of his own

I completely understand John's need and desire to do something monumental and magnanimous. The thing is, I really don't want to give away my kidney. I feel ungenerous saying so, but frankly I have had enough medical procedures to last several lifetimes, and I'm not done yet.

I don't suppose anyone would even want my kidney or any of my other innards, or even my blood. I think having had cancer makes me a bad risk.

All I have to offer is my story—this book. It is my homage to the importance of family and friends and community and good fortune. It is my thank you to everybody who ran with me in the marathon of my life.

Tommy, for rising to the occasion, always. Micah, Amit and Safi, my reasons for fighting so hard. Gina and Vivian Rakoff, to whom I wish I could promise no more misadventures. Simon Rakoff, who I must say makes the best lasagna, and Zoe Zucker-Rakoff. David Rakoff, who is an exemplary caregiver, especially for a guy who lives on his own. Joyce and Seymour Bellman, for everything you did, particularly for the boys. Mitchell, Nicola, Emma, Noah and Abby Bellman-Hamer for the hat and scarf and socks that managed somehow to warm my heart as much as my neck, head and feet.

To the team of medical specialists to whom I owe my life: Wendy Brown, Claire Holloway, Mark Clemons, Jamie Shiner, Anne Blaire, Helen Marks and John Semple. And all the nurses, pharmacists and hospital staff who I do not have the privilege of knowing by name. A special thanks to cousin Tamara Shenkier, who answered all my crazy questions with the knowledge of an oncologist and the empathy of kin. And to Noga Freeman, who not only came over to monitor the home-care nurses and give me my weekly shots, but also brought beautiful baby Lee with her to feed my spirit.

To my healing circle who repeatedly surrounded me with love, I cannot say enough: Cathy Mallove and Martin Geffen, Kate Scowen and Grant Edmonds, Iris Nemani and Mike Biderman, Maureen and Dave Carter-Whitney, Audrey Kalman and Peter Tostevin, Susan Aharan, Adrienne Rosen and Myra White, Jane Angus, Angela Stukator, Claudia Skolnik and David Slater, Sally Thomas and John Fulford, Amy Jubas and Jonathan Bernstein, Sindy and David Preger, Shiphra Ginsberg and Stuart Lewis, Sam Goldstein, Annie Bunting and Bruce Ryder, Ian Sinclair and Loren Fantin, Mark O'Hara and Tim Bond, Jill Magen and Gary Lichtblau and Tracy Rumig and Steve Eichler (who I promised to thank as my lawyer, but whose friendship I value even more than his legal advice).

For everybody who brought meals and flowers and books and magazines and treats and gifts, or called or visited or took care of and fed our children, I am eternally grateful to each and every one of you (in no particular order): Valerie Laflamme and Geoff Cape, Elizabeth Rochon and Eric Dreyfuss, Elana and Dave Seligman, Lori and Uncle Sam Merson, Rael and Karen Merson, Michael and Cheryl Levick, Auntie Riva and Uncle Raymond Levick, Marvin and Julia Spritzer, Gene and

Mark Teeger, Kathy and Maurice Green, Jean Marlow, Dionie Ibon, Linda and Dani Benishai, Michael and Carol Bain, Joyce Young, Ruth Mandel, Marla Fine and Bob Gagne, Kevin McMahon, Alejandra Priego and Neil Gardiner, Candy Girling and Aaron Davis, Andrea Bellman and Norm Melamed, Edith and Maurice Bellman, Lorna Rosenstein, Ann Rosenfield, Sarah Doyle, Deborah and Corrado Virginella, Caroline and Peter Harvey, Heidi Coleman and Glenn Hilke, Michele Coleman and Jaimie Shapiro, Adele and Len Wechsler, Avril Benoit and Allan Novak, Diane Pitblado and Mark Wilson, Brenda and Peter Simon, Carolyn Murphy and Dan Dunsky, Esther Levin, Christine Martin, Lise Fournier and Chris Diorio, Cathy Tafler and Doug Rylett, Jackie Silverberg, Donna Gray and Pat Thompson, Shawn and Noga Freeman, Karen Gold, Suzie Stewart, Nancy Markle and Keith Watson, Joanne and Vez Pajkovik, Vanessa Ring and John Nabereznyj, Blume and Isaac Sakinofsky, Pam and Mark Evans, Nina-Marie and Paul Lister, Jenny Knox, Scott Williamson and Leslie Peck, Shima and Todd Warren, Jacque and Tom Friedland, Scott Dammerman, Lynn Horton and John Gregory, Karen Beattie and Louis Sokolov, Karen White and Andrew Malcolm, Jennifer Baichwal and Nick DePencier, Meryl and Jeff Rosenthal, Heather Sloman and Phil Reese, Val and Leon Sloman, Valerie McDonald and Bruce Stratton,

Laurie and John Zinkand-Selles, Phil Stilman and Ruthie Torchinsky, Anne Stilman and Greg Ioannou, Jamie and Danielle Bush, Fay Faraday and Jim Lebans, Christina McCarthy, Sue Baker, Mina Mastromarco, Debbie and Chris Albertane, Sondra Vandervaart and Mike Lapenna, Lori and Joel Waldman, Carla Sorbara and Sol Korngold, Chella Tingley and Terry Drummond, Taisa and Brendan Dorney, Lindsey Tashlin, John Samuels, Sherry Kulman, Louise Gwynn, Debbie Paulino, Ginny Brett, Beryl Tsang, Mary Anne Janecki, Joy Schreiber, Alex and Simmy Davids, Jordanna and Rob Geist, Elisa Shenkier, Edith and Leonard Coleman, Auntie Lorna and Uncle Toffee Katz, Phyllis Kessler and Ayhan Sumer, Harriet and Marcel Grunwald, Peter Howard, Mark and Corinne Greenberg, Dov and Freidja Marmur, Jen Green and Michael Smolash, Steven and Faye Rakoff, Dovie Rakoff and Andrea Frankel, Julian Sakinofsky, Ruth and Danny Silver, Ruth and Doug Wilansky, Joy Schreiber, Hope Sealey, Lauren and Frida Kaminer, and Rhona and Ralph Hirschowitz. And Jean and Raziel Gershater, whose journeys ended far too soon.

Thanks to the women of my writing group for all of their invaluable feedback and for encouraging me to submit my work for publication: Valerie McDonald, Lynn Horton, Shila Desai, Anita Morris and Karen Laurence. (Note: remember these names. This won't be the last time you'll see them in print.)

Thanks to the women of Body & Soul for helping me find the confidence to believe that others might be interested in my stories: Judith Thompson, Rhonda Tepper, Lois Fine, Francine Grainger, Jeannine Boucher, Glenda Klassen, Judy Wark, Pauline Patten, Ann Marie Hasley, Janice Kulyk Keefer, Gloria Schmed-Scott, Barbie Nichol, Maria Costa and Brenda Surminski.

To my editor Pamela Murray, I thank you for your clarity and your patience in dealing with a newbie author. Thanks, too, to Allyson Latta and Liba Berry for copyediting and proofreading the book. And to Scott Sellers, Anne Collins and all the people at Random House who had the courage to take a chance on me, I am eternally in your debt.

To Kevin Kelly for his inordinate patience and insightful vision.

And for all the children, teenagers and young adults in my life:

Thank you, thank you, thank you.

Can I stop shutting up yet?

{ 213 }

Auntie Lorna's Baked Matzo Balls

Auntie Lorna would painstakingly fill each delicious lump of divinely dense yumminess with fried onions, whereas I simply mix the fried onions into the batter. I like to bake them in mini muffin tins (kind of like Jewish Yorkshire puddings).

For the batter I've provided basic proportions, though I have never in my life made only two eggs' worth of matzo balls. I usually factor about half an egg per person, rounding up of course and then just to be sure there will be enough add two more.

Onions

Use at least one medium onion or more (never less) for every egg.

Chop and fry onions slowly on low heat until beautifully caramelized. Traditionally this would be done in chicken fat, but I use olive oil. Allow the onions to cool.

Batter (basic proportions)

2 eggs

2 tablespoons oil or chicken fat

1/2 cup matzo meal

1 teaspoon salt

2 tablespoons soup or water

Lightly scramble eggs and oil together. Mix with matzo meal and salt until paste-like. Add water and stir out any lumps. Add generous amount of caramelized onions and stir into batter. Refrigerate for an hour or more.

Spoon ragged-edged lumps into greased mini muffin tins and bake at 350 degrees Fahrenheit until golden brown, about 12 to 15 minutes.

Try to wait till they cool before eating them.

RUTH RAKOFF was born in Montreal. She has had many careers, filled countless volunteer roles and dabbled in many of the arts. Currently she is working on her first novel. She lives in Toronto, where she cooks dinner every night for her husband and three sons.